Intermittent Fasting For Women After 50

The Beginner's Guide For Aging Women To Lose Weight, Detox The Body, Have Increased Energy And Start The Journey Towards Health And Longevity

MARTHA KIRBY

Thank you for choosing this book, I care about my readers' opinions, so I would love, once I read it, to get feedback and I kindly ask you to leave me a small review on Amazon.

Martha Kirby

Table of Contents

Introduction **5**

Chapter 1: Basics of Intermittent Fasting **7**

    1.1 What Is Intermittent Fasting and How it Started? 7

    1.2 The Science Behind Intermittent Fasting 10

    1.3 Various Intermittent Fasting Protocols 13

    1.4 Health Benefits of Intermittent Fasting 18

    1.5 Who Is IF Not Good For? 22

    1.6 Common Myths about IF 25

    1.7 Intermittent Fasting FAQs 28

Chapter 2: Intermittent Fasting for Women Over 50 .... **32**

    2.1 The Science Behind Menopause and Weight Gain 32

    2.2 How Men vs. Women Respond to IF? 34

    2.3 How IF Affects Female Hormones? 36

    2.4 Post-Menopausal Benefits of Intermittent Fasting 38

    2.5 Is Intermittent Fasting Safe for Older Women? 40

    2.6 Helpful Tips for Older Women Starting IF 42

Chapter 3: A Guide to Intermittent Fasting and Food **46**

    3.1 What To Eat And Avoid On IF Diet? 46

    3.2 Best Supplements for Intermittent Fasting 51

    3.3 Best Foods to Break Your Fast 53

Chapter 4: Get Started With Intermittent Fasting **56**

    4.1 Your 4-week Intermittent Fasting Plan 56

    4.2 Tasty and Healthy Breakfast Recipes 91

    4.3 Tasty and Healthy Lunch Recipes 96

    4.4 Tasty and Healthy Dinner Recipes 101

    4.5 Tasty and Healthy Dessert Recipes 106

    4.6 Tasty and Healthy Snacks Recipes 110

Conclusion **115**

Introduction

First and foremost, thank you for purchasing INTERMITTENT FASTING FOR WOMEN AFTER 50. Today is the day that you start to take charge of your life for the better, and it's is going to change your life and health forever. An intermittent fasting lifestyle for women after 50 always works like a miracle for weight loss, longevity, and overall vibrant health. If you follow this plan perfectly, it's going to be like the elixir of youth for you.

This book will teach you everything you need to know about intermittent fasting for older women. This book will teach you everything you need to know about intermittent fasting, including what it is, how it functions, and how to tailor it to your specific needs as a woman after 50. The intermittent fasting plan is amongst the most popular strategies to reduce weight since it is not restricting and also promotes a lifestyle shift.

All humans have an inborn tendency to fast, which makes it easier to implement intermittent fasting in our everyday routines. In reality, as you get adjusted to your new intermittent fasting lifestyle, you'll notice that you don't consume as much as you believe you do or have to. Fasting will not only help you reduce weight, but it will also help you satisfy your food requirements, battle illnesses, and enjoy a balanced lifestyle. Fasting was always and still continues to be an effective method to cleanse or purge the body off of chemicals and extra weight. Scientific research on the efficacy of intermittent fasting has found that it helps you to improve mental wellbeing and reduce health-related issues. The advantages of intermittent fasting are as many as the stars in the sky. And this book will explore it all in-depth, including a planned schedule, tips, and recipes.

Remember to set your goals and objectives to reach success when you first begin intermittent fasting. This can be particularly useful during extended fasts, as you may feel temporary hunger that will pass after your body adjusts to the new eating plan. You'll see that this book discusses a wide range of topics related to intermittent fasting; giving you all the information you need to get started. This book also debunks the widespread belief that breakfast is an essential meal of the day and can thus not be missed. Furthermore, nutritionists would advise you to take enough tiny meals throughout the day in order to remain well, but the intermittent fasting plan opposes this advice. Various observational experiments have shown that you can potentially miss breakfast, which supports the evidence behind intermittent fasting.

In this book, we'll talk about a variety of topics starting from the basics of what intermittent fasting s and how it works, its benefits, common myths surrounding it, and FAQs. Then, we'll move on to discussing IF with regards to women over 50. The book will highlight the science behind menopause and why women gain weight around this time. Then, we'll dive into the impact of IF on female hormones and how it can reduce the discomfort associated with menopause. The next chapter will contain everything you need to know about IF and food. The chapter will enlist the best foods to eat and stay away from on an intermittent fasting plan, along with the best foods that you can eat to break your fast. Finally, the book will end with a chapter containing a 4-week IF plan and healthy recipes from breakfast to dinner and snacks.

Chapter 1: Basics of Intermittent Fasting

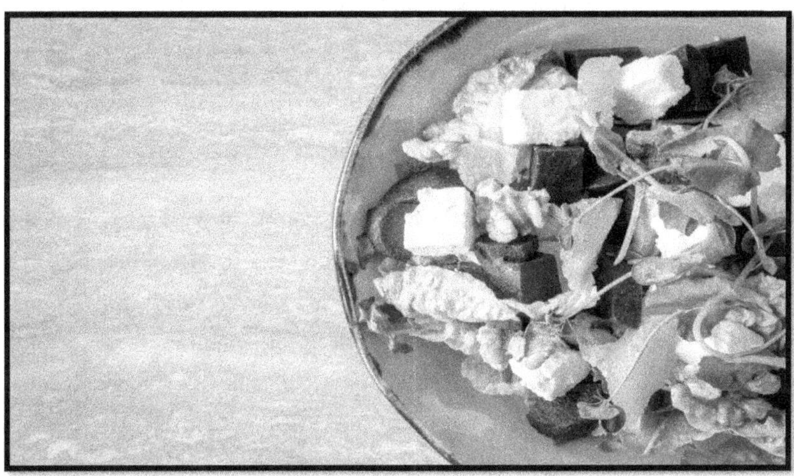

The topic of intermittent fasting (IF) is gaining a lot of traction these days in the health, fitness, and longevity circles. If you're new to the concept, this chapter contains all the necessary information you need to know about IF so that you can start a healthy and vibrant life once and for all. We'll start off with the basics of what IF is and what are its origins. Then, we'll dive into the actual evidence-based science behind this seemingly-magical method of weight loss. Then, once you've gained enough understanding of the concept of fasting, we'll talk about the various protocols you can follow as per your health needs and comfort level. The chapter will also contain a subsection on all the very many health benefits of IF, from weight loss to skin health to cancer prevention and much more. Furthermore, we'll also learn about the individuals who shouldn't do IF. Lastly, some widespread IF myths will be debunked, and FAQs will be answered.

1.1 What Is Intermittent Fasting and How it Started?

Rather than a conventional diet, intermittent fasting is a way of feeding. An intermittent fasting diet emphasizes what you eat rather than what you eat, while a conventional diet emphasizes when you eat. You alternate through cycles of extreme or full-calorie reduction (in other words, fasting) and phases of healthier eating in this eating style. The duration of these calorie-restricted and healthy-eating cycles varies as per personal preference.

Intermittent fasting is a lifestyle that alternates between periods of fasting (either no food or a substantial decrease in calories) and periods of uncontrolled feeding. It is advised to improve indicators of wellbeing that are linked to diabetes, such as cholesterol and triglyceride levels, as well as to alter body structure by losing body fat and weight. Traditional fast, as defined in sacred texts by Plato, Aristotle, and religious communities, is a common practice used for medical or religious gain. Fasting usually involves abstaining from food and drink for a period of time, varying from 12 hours to one week. It could necessitate full withdrawal or only enable a limited variety of nutrients and drink.

In the most basic form, fasting entails abstinence for a couple of days or a span of time and eventually returning to regular feeding. Intermittent fasting is a common diet these days, but it wouldn't have the same characteristics as a traditional diet! Like every other lifestyle, you consume a certain way and in a certain order, with a checklist of things to minimize and avoid. When it comes to intermittent fasting, there are no fast and quick rules for what foods to consume and what foods to avoid. Fasting often would not necessitate sticking to a rigid timetable when you cannot indulge!

Anyone, at any moment, will practice intermittent fasting. It does not stipulate that you would do it for a week, a month, or six months. You should do that as much as you want, because if you enjoy it if the body understands the way of eating and benefits you, you can almost certainly follow the diet. There really is no risk about someone quitting in the first week. There are no health consequences.

You have access to food; however, you prefer not to consume it. This may be over any length of time, from a few hours to a few days, or sometimes a week or more if medical supervision is provided. You can start a quick whenever you want, and you can finish it whenever you want. Intermittent fasting is where you don't feed for a long period of time. For e.g., you might fast for 12-14 hours from dinner to breakfast the following day. Fasting can be deemed a part of daily life in this way.

In the most simplistic form, fasting is a method of eating that is scheduled. Unlike most regimes, intermittent fasting depends solely on the timing of the meals. It focuses on giving the body the requisite rest time in between meals while also the output of accumulated fat as the body's primary fuel supply. Intermittent fasting may be customized to the own requirements and is usually done on a weekly or even regular basis.

Why is it appropriate to alter your dietary habits? Most importantly, it's a smart way to get slim without being on a fad diet or severely restricting your food intake. In reality, when you first begin intermittent fasting, you'll aim to maintain your calorie intake steadily. The majority of people consume larger portions in a shorter amount of time. Intermittent starvation is often a healthy way to maintain muscle strength when losing weight. Having said that, the primary motivation for people to pursue intermittent fasting is to lose some weight. Perhaps notably, since it takes relatively little lifestyle adjustment, intermittent fasting is among the best methods people have for losing weight while maintaining a healthy diet. This is a positive thing because it implies intermittent fasting meets the definition of "easy enough to perform, but significant enough to make a difference." The majority of people fast intermittently each night while sleeping. Our bodies are in a fasting period for 10–14 hours while they are at rest, which corresponds to the sleep cycle. This alignment, according to researchers, is crucial for maximum wellbeing.

History of Intermittent Fasting

Fasting isn't a modern concept. It has been performed since the beginning of human history. In actuality, the human species is programmed to do fasting. The hunter-gatherer people had a lot of food to stock, and due to shortages, they would often go hungry. As a result, they had the capacity to survive for extended stretches of time without eating, which is basically abstinence. Fasting has a religious component for Muslims and Christians both. Intermittent fasting is used by people all around the world to shed weight. Most people see it as a risk, and evidence has proven that intermittent fasting will help you lose weight. Some people fast intermittently merely to save time; they don't live to consume food, but they eat to thrive! They are content if they can miss meals, and intermittent fasting makes missing meals helpful. IF dieting is a common way for certain people to stay healthy and active. According to studies, individuals who fast for at least two times a week are more involved in other aspects of their lives, sleep well at night, and are happier. Intermittent fasting, too, is practiced in religion. People in Islam fast for a month and come out looking happier than they do in the past. Intermittent fasting is practiced in Buddhism, Hinduism, Catholicism, and by certain individuals to pay homage to their maker and to become religiously and physically pure.

Dr. Michael Mosley, on the other hand, popularized the new trend of intermittent fasting diets. Intermittent fasting has been gaining popularity, with an increasing number of citizens adopting it. The science underlying intermittent fasting is explained by Dr. Mosley. He, on the other hand, credits intermittent fasting's effectiveness and acceptance to the idea that it is mostly therapeutic and gives you healthier eating habits. That is after you've been used to consuming veggies and lean protein, you'll begin to desire it when you're starving.

1.2 The Science Behind Intermittent Fasting

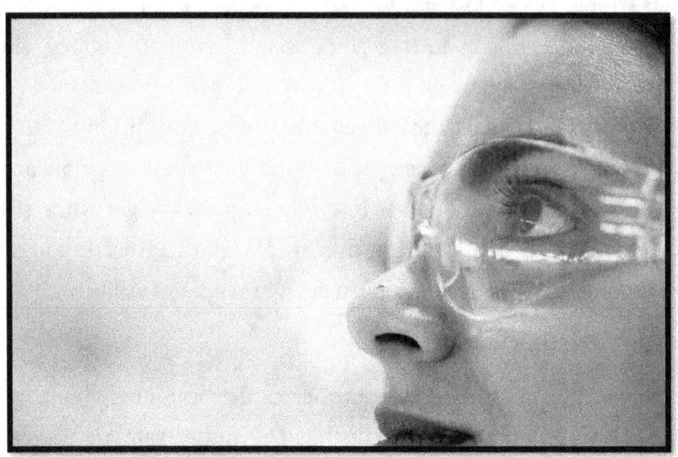

Intermittent fasting, at the most basic level, essentially helps the body to utilize its surplus resources by consuming excess body fat. It's crucial to remember that this is natural, and humans have adapted to be able to fast for limited times – days or hours – without experiencing negative health effects. An excess number of calories is usually accumulated in the form of body fat. Your body would actually "consume" its very own fat for fuel if you don't eat. Life is just about finding the right mix. The yin or the yang, the positive and the bad. The same is so when it comes to food and abstinence. Overall, fasting is just the opposite of feeding. People are fasting when they're not consuming. The following is how it works:

When we feed, we provide more nutritional calories than we would use right now. Any of this fuel would have to be saved for later. Insulin is a hormone that helps the body retain energy from food. When we feed, our insulin levels increase, assisting us in storing additional energy in 2 ways. Carbs are glucose broken down into glucose (sugar) units that can be joined together to form glycogen, which is then retained in the liver or muscle.

However, there is a finite amount of storage capacity for sugars, and when the cap is hit, the liver begins to convert the extra glucose to fat. De-novo lipogenesis (literally "making fresh fat") is the name given to this method. The liver stores some of the freshly produced fat, although the majority of it is distributed to other fatty tissue in the body. Although this is a more challenging task, the amount of fat that can be generated is almost limitless.

In our bodies, we have two important energy storage processes. One is simple to access but has minimal storage capacity (glycogen), while the other is more complex to use but has nearly infinite storage capacity (lipids). If we don't feed, the mechanism reverses. Insulin levels drop, indicating the body to begin consuming stored energy since food is no longer accessible. Since sugar levels are dropping, the liver must now draw glucose from inventory to use for fuel.

Glucose is the most readily available source of energy. To supply sugar to the body's other cells; it is decomposed into sugar molecules. This will last for 24-36 hours and have sufficient energy to meet much of the body's needs. Afterward, the body's primary source of nutrition would be the fat breakdown.

So there are only two conditions in which the body may exist: fed and fasted. We are either storing food resources (increasing stores) or consuming stored energy (burning stored energy) (decreasing stores). It's either this or that. There can be no net weight difference if feeding and abstinence are matched. We waste nearly half of our life in the fed condition whether we start feeding as soon as we get out of bed and don't pause before we go to sleep. We may accumulate weight over time because we haven't given our bodies enough energy to destroy stored food fuel. We will just need to maximize the period of time we spend utilizing energy from food to regain equilibrium or lose weight. Intermittent fasting is what it's called.

Intermittent fasting, in turn, enables the body to utilize the remaining fat. What's essential to remember is that there's nothing incorrect with it. That is the way our beings are made. That's what dogs, mice, bears, and wolves do. That's what people do. Your body can constantly utilize the new food resources if you feed every 2 hours, which is frequently advised. It might not be enough to expend much if any, body fat. It's possible that you're simply accumulating fat. It's possible that the body is storing it until a moment when you won't be able to feed. If this occurs, you are out of control. You're missing out on intermittent fasting.

Most hormones in the body are affected by fasting, like the appetite hormones ghrelin and leptin. Intermittent fasting, as previously mentioned, lowers ghrelin levels and can aid weight loss. Intermittent fasting may help with weight loss by lowering blood glucose and insulin levels, lowering LDL ("bad") cholesterol level triglyceride levels and reducing inflammation. It's worth noting, however, that the majority of research into how intermittent fasting impacts body chemistry has been conducted on males.

Feeding Vs. Fasting – The Trouble with the Modern Age

Human beings did not grow to consume several little meals during the day and evening. Humans, on the other hand, also learned to cope with daily fasts: We survived on hunting and collecting until the advent of agriculture about 12,000 years ago, and we mostly had to do so with hungry bellies. We are programmed to practice intermittent fasting on a regular basis. Furthermore, people are feeding during periods of the day that they may have been sleeping in the past. For millennia, our nighttime fasting period actually began even sooner than it does now because late-night television and other electrically powered entertainments (such as Zoom sessions) encourage us to sit up late and snack late.

To comprehend how intermittent fasting contributes to fat loss, we must first comprehend the distinction between the fed and fasted states. When the body digests and absorbs food, it is in a fed condition. The fed condition usually begins when you start feeding and lasts 3 to 5 hours as your system digests and consumes the nutrition you just consumed. Since your insulin levels are elevated while you're in the fed state, it's difficult for your body to burn fat.

During that time period, the body enters a condition recognized as the post-absorptive condition, which is simply a sophisticated way of suggesting that it isn't absorbing a meal. The post-absorptive condition continues before you reach the fasted state, which is 8 to 12 hours from your last meal. Since the insulin levels are poor, it is much simpler for your body to lose fat while you have fasted.

Fasting allows the body to metabolize fat that was previously unavailable, mostly during the eating state. The bodies are rarely in this fat-burning condition, and we don't reach the fasted condition before 12 hours from our last meal. This is one of the explanations that many people who begin intermittent fasting lose weight without altering their diet, amount of food consumed, or frequency of exercise. Fasting induces a fat-burning condition in your body that you seldom achieve with a regular feeding routine.

1.3 Various Intermittent Fasting Protocols

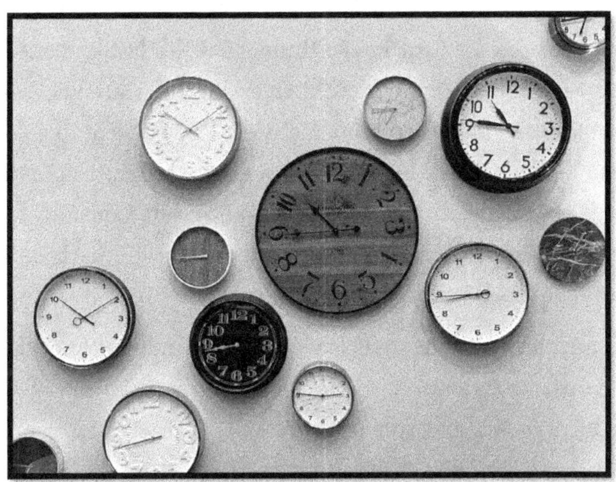

Although intermittent fasting has no limitations, there are a few methodological discrepancies between the different types. There are several common approaches to the diet. Many of the techniques are effective and known to assist you in achieving your objectives of gaining weight, becoming more energized and active, reducing exhaustion, combating overeating, achieving a youthful look, enhancing digestion, and combating a variety of diseases. Fasting, though, is not a one-size-fits-all method. That principle would not apply to intermittent fasting. Intermittent fasting is adaptable, and since no two bodies work in the same manner, intermittent fasting will benefit you in a variety of ways. No one will promise that one strategy would perform better for you than the others before you test each one for yourself. You must determine which one fits well for you after testing them out. And you are more comfortable with the body. Just because a technique works with someone else does not imply it would work with you. To find the perfect match, you must just go and test it out for yourself.

The various types of fasting protocols are mentioned below.

1. 20:4 Fast (aka The Warrior Diet)

Simply put, the diet entails a 20-hour fast accompanied by a 4-hour eating time frame as the name suggests; it is based on the dietary patterns of ancient fighters, who definitely did not consume several meals each day. As per the source, warriors in societies spanning from Roman knights to the Spartan aristocracy ate one to main servings a day: a big dinner in the evenings and (occasionally) a small breakfast in the morning. Since the plan is based around this sort of eating routine, it's worth mentioning that it's often blamed for being not "real" IF.

Furthermore, the diet provides for light intake throughout the fasting period of the day. You needed/wanted; you'd be able to consume a few servings of fresh fruits and vegetables, as well as only several portions of meat (protein powders included). This is kept to a minimum. Warrior dieting, on the other hand, is not fasting, according to some diet enthusiasts. As a result, you won't reap any of the rewards of extended fasting. A 20-hour quick works similarly to a 24-hour fast in that it helps you to enjoy the hormonal benefits of elevated growth hormone. And, as with any fasting, it can lead to a reduction in calorie consumption.

The advantage of this method of abstinence is that you usually only consume one big meal, so the composition of the meal isn't as essential as you would believe; as far as you have enough nutrition, you could eat unhealthier items and still perform well. Furthermore, eating only one meal simplifies life, and less thought implies fewer mistakes.

Since it's named the warrior diet, you can feed the same way our ancestral warriors did: "organic food." You can only consume unprocessed foods; in other words, "whole food" is the direction to go for this approach. The Warrior Diet strategy is somewhat close to the "paleo" dietary options.

2. 16/8 Fasting (aka LeanGains)

It's a ritual fasting process that involves going hungry for 16 hours and only eating for the next 8 hours. Users will consume as many (or as few) meals as they choose during this period, with three meals being one of the most common variant. This technique was coined by fitness specialist Martin Berkhan as the LeanGains protocol. The 16/8 intermittent fasting process entails abstaining from food for 16 hours and only allowing yourself to feed for the following 8 hours. Muslims practice this form of fasting during Ramadan, beginning their fast at sunrise and ending it at sunset. They fast for 30 days and emerge, feeling cleansed and energized. Everybody who is hesitant or concerned for their wellbeing need not be scared. Of course, you don't have to perform a month of 16/8 extended fasting; they're doing so for religious reasons. You should do that as much as you like as long as your digestive system is capable of supporting it.

If you consider it, you've actually done a 16/8 easy at some point in your life. Consider the times you had a late dinner at 7 p.m. and ended up at midday or awoke late and missed breakfast. That way, you've already abstained from food for 16 hours without even realizing it! Now, if you can manage it unconsciously, you could do it as you make the deliberate choice to go on a rules-free, low-calorie diet!

The 16/8 approach is the most common type of Intermittent Fasting for those who exercise for beauty and body enhancement since it was designed explicitly with fitness in mind and includes detailed post-workout tips and guidelines. The 16/8 approach is unique in that it provides for advanced hormone management in addition to many of the advantages associated with other forms of Intermittent Fasting. Although twenty-four-hour fast or alternate-day fasting will have these advantages, they are not recommended for everyday use, while 16/8 is. This ensures that the GH levels can rise on a regular basis, further amplifying the symptoms.

This IF system can be used as much as you'd like, or sometimes once a week or two times a week, depending on your preferences. It may take several days to find out the best feeding and fasting periods for this process, particularly if you're really busy or if you awaken starving for breakfast. For those people who like to pursue intermittent fasting for the very first time, this is a better option.

3. 24-Hour Fasting (Eat. Stop. Eat method)

This mechanism is very straightforward. You must abstain from food for a total of 24 hours. There is nothing you can consume for 24 hours here in these 24 hours. Of necessity, you can remain hydrated by drinking water. When you're fasting, it's important to remain well-hydrated. You're doing intermittent fasting to boost your fitness. However, dehydration can occur. While you're on a juice soon, you need to be especially alert. You must consume plenty of water in order to remain well hydrated. Four days with nothing but herbal tea would have little to no effect on the person who has been dieting for twenty-four hours, although on the other hand, after a twenty-four-hour water fast, a person might be hungry for just four or five days. What would the diet do then? Digestive complications can occur this way. Be on your guard for such stuff.

The fitness guru Brad Pilon pioneered this approach, which has been very famous for several years. And during short, liquids such as water, caffeine, as well as other low-calorie drinks are tolerated, but food items are not. Brad Pilon and his work called "Eat-Stop-Eat," which is the ultimate book on this type of fasting, is unavoidable when discussing 24-hour fasts. Aside from the caloric manipulation, this method of fasting is extremely effective due to the impact it has on the general biochemical condition. When we speak about fasting, we're talking about two chemicals in particular: insulin and growth hormone. When it comes to insulin, it appears that the little you consume, the less insulin you create. Evidently, this is not shocking. It's also less shocking that this will result in weight loss, given how impossible it is to burn calories while insulin levels are consistently raised. As a result, even though you consume the same ingredients in the very same proportions, if you eat less frequently, you'll have less insulin problems.

If you are looking at your schedule for something fresh, make sure to do some intensive sightseeing the day before the deadline. Most people will take more time to get used to the idea of intermittent fasting, so don't expect immediate results. Several individuals have managed to keep a 24-hour day a week schedule for many years; it's certainly not difficult for you to do so. Physically, anorexic individuals will normally last for 24 hours. A newcomer is likely to become extremely irritable in the course. You can try intermittent fasting before you decide to use other forms of fasting.

4. 5:2 fasting

If the "no food" lifestyle doesn't fit you, try the 5:2 approach. This diet differs from the most other alternate day fasting methods in that you eat 500 calories on two days a week and eat normally the other five days. There is a greater need for 5:2 fasting in order to maintain weight and for five days while following a 500-600 calorie limit for two days. No one has to tell you what to eat or what to drink as long as it fits inside the calorie range of 500-600. Calorie needs vary in males and females, resulting in women having 500 kcal constraints and men having 600 kcal constraints. Each day's schedule may be planned by the person. While you are at your employment, you can successfully handle the additional days. So, for one week, Wednesday and Sunday, you have free choice, and the other week you must comply. That may be on any two non-consecutive days of the week. In order to stay slim, allow oneself to eat only twice a day. Bulk up on nutritious foods to ensure you don't consume more calories. It is also known as Michael Mosley's Fast diet.

You may feed on every day, excluding Tuesdays and Fridays. For both of these two days, you prepare two 250 calorie meals for females and one extra for males. It is said that the fast days should be mixed evenly. Offer your body a minimum of one day between those fasting days for a break. You can select two days of abstinence, as far as there is one non-fasting day between them (e.g., Mondays and Weds). If you are not going to abstain, then make sure you consume the very same quantity of food on non-fasting times.

5. Alternate Day Fasting

This is also daunting since it demands that one fast the whole day before moving on to the regular eating routine. Then keep abstinence for the entire next day. This approach is well suited for those who have prior experience of intermittent fasting. This diet pattern entails rotating periods of fasting and normal feeding. It is equivalent to the two- or three-day fast.

Alternative day fasting involves several extended fasting times during the week. For instance, you will consume the food on Monday evening and abstain from food till Tuesday. On Wednesday, you will begin a 24-hour fast following supper. This improves your regularity while still helping you to maintain a steady food supply. The bonus of alternating day fast is that it allows you to stay in the fasted condition for a prolonged period of time. Speculatively, this will boost the fasting effects.

In addition, training oneself to consume less regularly may be one of the most difficult aspects of intermittent fasting. You may be free to partake in a meal every now and again, but the process is challenging and demanding. It is discovered that the bulk of folks who attempt IF wind up gaining more weight, while a few portions are eliminated every week.

6. 12:12 fasting

This is yet another practical choice for those who are new to prolonged fasting. You will have the option to fast for 12 hours before eating for the next 12 hours. This form of fasting is simple and therefore does not trigger food cravings. Often participants aren't really aware that they are acting in a different way. This form of fasting may be tried by either missing breakfast or dinner. If you follow this tool, it's so much simpler to fast nearly every day.

7. 18:6 fasting

For several people who want to gradually improve the advantages of a lengthy fast, this could be the second move after 16:8. When the feeding window is shortened by 2 hours, from 8 to 6, the number of meals consumed during that time span increased be limited. If you work a normal 9-to-5 job, a 6-hour window might start at 7 a.m. and finish following brunch or an afternoon treat, from 1 p.m. to 7 a.m. the next morning.

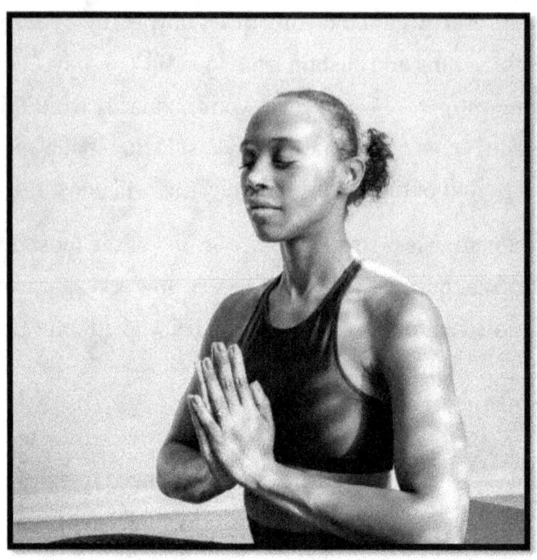

A variety of studies have shown that intermittent fasting has significant mental and physical health effects. When you start fasting for weight reduction, you'll reap the following benefits:

1. Weight Loss

Intermittent eating is one of the most effective ways to burn fat quickly. Through intermittent fasting, fat burning occurs as a consequence of being in a calorie-deficient condition, which causes fat loss. In research on cattle, it was discovered that intermittent abstinence for up to 16 weeks would help prevent overweight, with effects visible in as little as five weeks. Intermittent fasting, according to science, helps to activate metabolic rate while also assisting in fat burning by the production of body heat. The insulin levels would be down while you're fasting. Glucose is broken down into glucose, which the cells use for nutrition, or they are converted into fat, which the body stores for future use. When you don't eat, the insulin levels are down. As a result, when you fast, your insulin is going to be poor, causing your cells to draw carbohydrates from stored fat for energy. As this step is replicated many times, weight reduction occurs. Intermittent eating seems to be a successful weight-loss technique, according to the majority of studies. Since you'll more likely be consuming fewer calories and nutrients, your body can mostly depend on fat reserves for nutrition, resulting in massive weight loss.

2. Insulin Resistance Prevention

When you feed, the liver breaks down the food into glucose, which is then sent to the cells by the bloodstream. To work properly, your cells depend on carbohydrates as a fuel source. Insulin is a chemical that causes glucose to be absorbed by cells. Insulin is released while you feed, prompting the cells to consume glucose. The cells efficiently obtain fuel as they receive glucose. This isn't always the case, however. In certain cases, the interaction between insulin and the organs breaks down, causing the glucose to be retained as fat instead of being received by the cells. Insulin resistance is the term for this condition. In other words, when the amount of insulin released increases, the cells will not react by obtaining glucose. Insulin resistance can be induced by a variety of factors, but the pancreas can only generate so much insulin until it becomes exhausted, resulting in insulin deficiency and diabetes. Once it occurs, you'll be drained, chilly, and miserable all of the time. This tolerance is determined not just by insulin levels but also by persistence. Intermittent fasting is a simple and effective way to improve insulin sensitivity. Your body enters ketosis as usable glucose and glycogen, which is accumulated glucose, are burned. Ketones are used to provide fuel.

3. Reduced Inflammation and Oxidative Stress

Most chronic illnesses and aging are preceded by oxidative damage. It includes reactive molecules such as free - radical reacting with and damaging certain molecules such as DNA and protein. Fasting improves the body's susceptibility to oxidative damage, according to many findings. Furthermore, intermittent fasting aids in the battle against inflammation, which is a popular cause of disease, especially when the body is capable of autophagy.

4. Cancer Prevention

Cancer is a disorder under which the unregulated proliferation of cells is manifested. Fasting has been shown in studies to have a variety of metabolic effects, including a lower incidence of cancer. Fasting has also been shown to reduce some of the side effects of chemotherapy in cancer patients. It's worth noting that much of these trials have been conducted on animals; therefore, further human research is needed.

5. Improved Cellular Repair

When you fast for a prolonged amount of time, the body's cells start a waste disposal mechanism called autophagy. This mechanism entails not just tearing down but also detoxifying damaged and fragmented proteins that build up in cells over time. Enhanced autophagy may defend against a variety of diseases, including Alzheimer's disease. Intermittent fasting enhances autophagy, which is a crucial detoxification mechanism in the body that helps to flush out dead cells. To put it another way, taking a break from food and metabolism allows the body to regenerate and rid itself of garbage that can speed up the aging process. According to a study published in 2019, time-restricted feeding, described as eating between the hours of 8 a.m. and 2 p.m., increases the activity of the autophagy genes and the protein which controls cell development. This was a limited survey, with just 11 people participating over the course of four days. Another research found that limiting food intake is a well-known way to improve autophagy, especially synaptic autophagy, which can have brain-protective effects. However, there were certain drawbacks to this research as well; it was conducted on mice rather than humans.

6. Better Sleep

If you've ever seemed like you've fallen into a comatose state after a large meal, you're aware that your diet will affect your alertness and drowsiness. As a consequence of adopting the IF diet; certain people seem to be able to rest easier. Sleep can be affected by IF and bedtimes. According to one hypothesis, IF controls the sleep cycle, which decides sleep schedules. You'll have an easier time falling asleep and waking up with a coordinated circadian rhythm. The other idea is that if you eat your last dinner early in the day, the food would have been digested by the point you reach the bed. As per the National Sleep Foundation, absorption is best achieved when you're standing up, and sleeping with a full belly can trigger acid reflux or heartburn, making it difficult to fall asleep.

Intermittent fasting often aids in the development of a healthy sleeping pattern. Fasting makes it impossible to sit up late at night, and keeping up through the night is harmful to one's wellbeing. The night is for resting because if you sit up late, you'll wake up with a horrible migraine or feel nauseous the rest of the day. Intermittent fasting allows you to go to bed and get up at the same time. This way, you'll still get stuff accomplished and be more involved.

7. Enhanced Brain Health

When one fasts, the brain hormone BDNF is enhanced. It's even possible that it's the source of new brain cell development. Intermittent fasting has been found to be effective in the treatment of Alzheimer's disease in several studies. Intermittent fasting improves cognitive functioning as well as providing a boost to brain capacity. Intermittent fasting increases the rate of brain-derived neurotropic factor (BDNF). This is a protein found in the brain that interacts with other areas of the brain that regulate thought, learning, and mental processes. The brain-derived neurotropic factor, too, is able to protect and enhance the connections between neurons. When you fast intermittently, the body enters a ketogenic condition, where ketones are used to convert excess weight to fuel. Ketones will also fuel the brain, resulting in increased cognitive efficiency, stamina, and alertness.

8. Decreased Cravings

We always have an unhealthy food craving, and whether you live by a fast food restaurant or drive by one on the way to work, you're in trouble! The scent emanating from the fast food place is enticing and difficult to avoid for any foodie. The unhealthy food cravings disappear entirely as you fast intermittently. Without really attempting to avoid it, you instinctively choose to move back from it. Since the body understands what is healthy for it, it refuses the taco bell craving.

9. Increased Metabolism

The human body isn't designed to have food available 24 hours a day, seven days a week. Our bodies adapted to survive times of deprivation, and researchers now understand that fasting causes the metabolic rate to change. When carbs (which are converted into sugars) aren't usable, the body switches to accumulated fats and ketones as a source of energy. Ketosis is the name for this method, and it's a really effective way of producing fuel. Eating stuff early in the day and increasing the nighttime fasting time will increase metabolism, as per Harvard Health.

10. Improved Blood Pressure

Physicians have long observed that individuals who frequently fast as a ritual cleansing have healthier bodies, causing others to speculate that prolonged fasting may be a tool for preventing myocardial infarction. The response wasn't obvious at first since religious fasters seem to live very healthier lifestyles in general; none are big drinkers or addicts, but avoidance (or mild use) of cigarettes and alcohol may have contributed to their good cardiovascular health. Intermittent fasting has also been found in medical research to be as successful as blood pressure meds in lowering blood pressure. Intermittent fasting has also been found in medical research to be as successful as blood pressure meds in lowering blood pressure. CCC

11. Improved Blood Sugar Levels

Scientists have understood for a long time that sustained fasting lowers blood glucose levels, but they couldn't tell whether the improvement was due to weight reduction or was due to the fasting phase itself. To find out, researchers measured the calorie requirements of several pre-diabetic men and required them to consume all meals between the hours of 8 a.m. and 2 p.m. for five weeks. While they did not lose fat, their blood glucose levels dramatically reduced.

12. Better Digestive Health

The cells of the digestive tract always remain busy. These cells function to the point that they are flushed away as excreta in certain cases. By ensuring that the body enters autophagy, you will fix these gastrointestinal cells with fasting. This eliminates the cellular debris and stimulates the immune system in the process. This is also true with a chronic intestinal immune reaction that may trigger gastrointestinal inflammation. Allowing them to relax helps them to regenerate and rebuild themselves. An extended night quick and autophagy will enable your gut to relax as well as recharge.

13. Promotes Longevity

Intermittent fasting has been shown to enable people to live longer lives. This idea goes back to the 1950s, when scientists found autophagy and its enormous capacity for deciding the overall quality of life. To put it another way, you don't need to consume a lot of nutrients to stay healthy; instead, focus on supporting the internal mechanism that recycles degraded cell pieces and destroys harmful body cells.

1.5 Who Is IF Not Good For?

While some people describe feeling more energized after intermittent fasting, others can feel fatigued, have trouble concentrating, or have low energy levels. This will have an effect on everyday performance. If you work in a job or do tasks that need a great deal of energy and focus, skipping breakfast may not be the best option for you. So, even though intermittent fasting is a common way of life for certain people, it isn't for everybody. Although fasting can be a safe option for many others, it may be risky for some people.

So who should abstain from intermittent fasting? Continue reading to learn more.

1. People with Digestive Issues

As if digestive problems weren't difficult enough to cope with, introducing a challenging eating regimen to the equation would just exacerbate the problem. If you already have digestive issues (such as IBS), IF can exacerbate your symptoms. Given the long fasting periods, IF may also trigger intestinal problems. Fasting can trigger bloating, heartburn, and stomach pain by disrupting the gastrointestinal system's regular functions. Large meals, which are sometimes needed for IF that need a lengthy fast, may trigger digestive problems. Those with Irritable bowel syndrome, who also have a vulnerable stomach, should be concerned about this.

2. People with a History of Eating Disorders

Intermittent starvation isn't a good idea while you're trying to rehab from maladaptive feeding. Those who have a propensity of anorexia nervosa or background of an eating disorder should choose to stop extended fasting. Fasting necessitates intervals of calorie reduction accompanied by cycles of greater food consumption. For those who deal with starving, binge eating, or other disturbing dietary habits, this may be particularly triggering. Under some situations, it's best to stop extended fasting entirely and adhere to a more regular eating schedule.

An eating condition, such as anorexia and bulimia or emotional eating may develop if erratic dietary habits and behavior are not handled. Intermittent restriction, according to experts, is not the best option for someone who has struggled with eating disorders or an addiction to food. In individuals with this experience, any approach that promotes restraint will lead to an unhealthy pattern. It's critical for everyone, but especially for anyone with this experience, to listen to their bodies and be aware of what makes them feel good psychologically and mentally.

3. Type 1 Diabetics

Fasting may be difficult for those with type 1 diabetes. The pancreas is unable to manufacture insulin, a chemical that transports glucose from the bloodstream to different cells in the body, including skeletal muscle, adipocytes, and even the liver. People with type 1 diabetes also need insulin doses in order to consume food without developing hyperglycemia, a condition in which there is so much glucose in the body. If you're diabetic and taking diabetes drugs, particularly insulin, you should never try intermittent fasting without first consulting a doctor and being closely watched. When fasting is paired with diabetes drugs, blood sugar levels may drop dangerously low. Anyone who suffers from low blood sugar can stop IF because they need to eat regularly to keep their blood sugar levels stable.

4. Pregnant or Breastfeeding Women

While you're pregnant, you ought to eat a nutritious (albeit calorie-dense) maternity diet to keep both the mother and the baby safe. You won't get it with fasting, unfortunately. Intermittent fasting is not recommended for people with serious conditions such as diabetes or cancer since it can result in low blood sugar, insufficient calorie consumption, and failure to satisfy nutritional requirements. Due to higher energy and nutrient requirements, this is also applicable for expectant mothers and nursing people. If you're pregnant, you'll need to feed frequently and in sufficient amounts to maintain your and your baby's wellbeing. Intermittent fasting's nature just does not provide for this. If you're planning to conceive, IF may not be the best option for you. IF has been attributed to reproductive problems, as well as improvements in menstruation, metabolic disturbances, and even pre-menopause in females.

5. Endurance Athletes

Nutrient timing is critical for athletic success, which will be difficult to do with an intermittent fasting schedule. Because of the extra calories expended, endurance activities necessitate higher calorie requirements. To regenerate tissue, replenish glycogen reserves, and retain electrolyte equilibrium, endurance exercise demands regular calorie intake and sufficient macros intake before, after, and all throughout an exercise or long training period. Intermittent fasting does not provide the consistent supply of nutritionally dense foods necessary for training, performance, and recovery. If you're planning on participating in an endurance race, you can stop intermittent fasting.

Likewise, if you're looking to add weight, you can ingest protein at various times during the day instead of trying to fit it all into a single feeding window. Most scientists believe that the body can't adequately synthesize upwards of 30-35 g of protein in a single session. As a consequence, any meat that is ingested but not used is usually stored as body fat.

6. People With Sleep Problems

Sleep is important for recovering and restoring muscles after exercise, promoting brain activity, and also preserving mental health. Going to bed hungry will make it difficult for your body and mind to rest and stay asleep because it triggers your mind to become vigilant, causing your body to become agitated. When you don't eat for many hours, the blood glucose levels decrease naturally, which may lead you to wake up feeling nervous in the dead of night. Disruptions in sleep can be dangerous to your health, particularly if they happen during the most important period of sleep, the rapid eye movement (REM) period. This phase is essential for remembering what you experienced throughout the day. In addition to interfering with weight control, insufficient sleep poses a safety concern in the role of brain ability and driving.

1.6 Common Myths about IF

Intermittent fasting has received a lot of attention recently. However, some people are still skeptical about whether it is good, effective, or even healthy. It's important to have the correct specifics whether you're contemplating or following intermittent fasting. You'll be more able to fast correctly if you have the evidence. And if you fast correctly, you'll be more likely to see the weight loss, consistent energy, and decreased hunger pangs that have rendered intermittent fasting so influential. There is a lot of misconception out there, apparently. Fasting misconceptions, on the other hand, are not founded on fact. Instead, they're built on gossip, speculation, and blind faith in old knowledge.

Let's dispel some of the more common misconceptions around intermittent fasting that you will make more educated choices around proper fasting as a health-improvement strategy.

1. You Cannot Eat Anything During Your Fasts

To begin with, taking out liquids is really not a good idea, so keep drinking water even though you're fasting intermittently. However, water should not be the only item you can eat throughout a fast. According to experts, the fast is theoretically over when the liver begins to digest the foods and beverages we consume. Many of the advantages of fasting come from the idea that you're extending the period you're in a low-insulin condition. This suggests that, while going beyond the established guidelines, consuming caffeine that does not induce insulin and eating a small amount of fat can be appropriate. Doctors also advocate drinking a cup of bulletproof morning coffee, remembering that the combination of coffee and butter incorporates healthier fats and sends the body into ketosis, or the process of switching from carbohydrates to ketones as the main fuel source (or fat). This will help you burn fat and speed up your system.

2. Fasting Causes Muscle Loss

Muscle mass tissue may be lost as a result of malnutrition. As a result, it seems fair to conclude that skipping breakfast would result in any muscular loss. However, research has demonstrated that fasting can help to preserve muscle mass as compared to traditional portion control. It has been proposed that a person must starve for 5 or more days in a row until some huge portion of muscle can be used for fuel. Muscle tissue is constantly broken down and replaced, and fasting may aid this phase by encouraging autophagy, or the clearance of old proteins in favor of newer ones, making it less likely to be weakened. Fasting paired with strength training has been shown to improve efficiency and muscle building in trained muscles in studies. Fasting increases growth hormones, which may justify some of this.

The truth is that just because you aren't consuming food, particularly protein, on a regular basis doesn't mean your body is in "catabolic" mode, as many people believe. Fasting breaks down muscle fibers for energy, only according to the theory that the body requires a regular flow of proteins to restore, sustain, and create muscle tissue.

Furthermore, a good portion of protein from the last meal previous to a 16-20 hour fast will definitely already be producing proteins by the moment you ended the fast again. It's not unusual for those doing intermittent fasting to eat a full meal of 70+ grams of slow-absorbing protein before starting again.

Bear in mind that prolonged fasting can result in muscle failure when "de novo gluconeogenesis" kicks in when muscle glycogen and amino acids are depleted; nevertheless, for people who fast intermittently and consume a big, nutritious meal until fasting again, none of these scenarios is likely to occur in 16-20 hours.

3. IF is Completely Safe For Everyone

Intermittent fasting is not recommended for the following people:

- Children and adolescents

- Those who are pregnant or nursing

- Those with eating disorders or a record of maladaptive eating patterns

Patients with diabetes or cardiovascular diseases should still seek medical advice before embarking on any new diet, according to experts.

4. Skipping Breakfast Makes You Gain Fat

Breakfast is sometimes misunderstood as the essential food of each day. Breakfast deprivation is generally thought to trigger increased appetite, hunger pangs, and excess weight. There was no weight disparity between those who consumed breakfast as well as those who didn't in a 16-week survey of 283 people who were obese or overweight. As a result, while there might be some human variability, breakfast does not have a significant impact on your weight. Most individuals profit from breakfast, but it is not needed for good health. There is little disparity in weight reduction between those who consume it and those who miss it, according to controlled trials.

5. IF is Not Natural!

Some people who are used to consuming three meals a day believe that skipping breakfast is the same as starvation, but experts say that fasting, particularly the 16/8 protocol, is completely normal. Humans are programmed to feed at certain times of the day. Since human beings are diurnal beings, our metabolic rates are set for feeding in the day.

6. It Will Deprive You Of Essential Nutrients

Participants of the abstinence groups did not show signs of starvation or nutritional loss in long-term medical studies. While breaking the fast, the value of the foods should be prioritized. Nutritional shortages may be avoided by eliminating packaged, poor foods and rising intake of nutritionally good, fresh foods. Finally, since fat-soluble vitamins are readily available, they have the ability to be distributed through the bloodstream from fat stores.

7. Fasting Causes Overeating

You'll be hungry after a fast. Many people believe that this hunger would lead to bingeing. The proof, on the other hand, refutes this worry. Attendees in most fasting trials are allowed to consume as much as they choose, a procedure known as ad-libitum eating. They feed to their hearts' content and still lose more weight. In reality, many intermittent fasting methods would cause you to consume fewer rather than more. As a result of the moderate calorie limit, you'll lose weight gradually without shutting down the metabolic processes.

Intermittent fasting has been shown to be a highly efficient weight loss strategy in several studies. Furthermore, there is no proof that skipping breakfast causes excess weight. It isn't to suggest that you won't add weight if you binge and overindulge through your munching times — you can. As a result of the physiological improvements that arise in the body, such as a decrease of insulin levels while also increasing metabolic rate, norepinephrine levels, and growth hormone concentrations, intermittent fasting is an effective method for weight control, allowing you to lose fat rather than accumulate it. The bottom line is that you shed pounds when you successfully build a calorie imbalance over time, through which you consume less energy and spend more. (If you flip this calculation on its head, you'll add weight.)

8. Alternate-Day Fasting is the Most Effective Strategy

There are many forms of intermittent fasting: Alternate day diet entails restricting calories to less than 500 a day, consumed all at once every other day. Meanwhile, 5:2 fasting entails eating normally for five days and heavily restrict food for the next two. Fasting for 16 hours and feeding

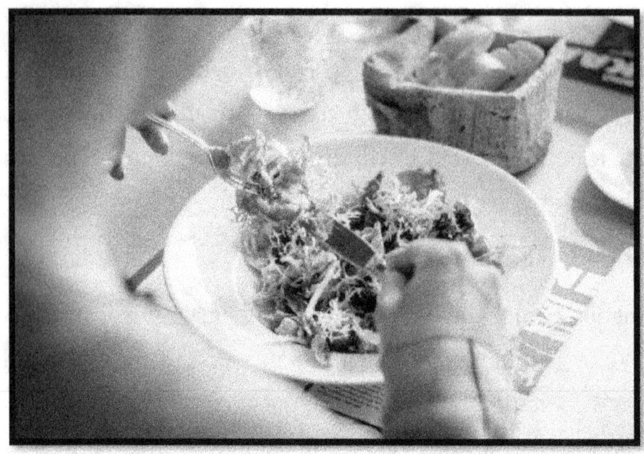

only over an eight-hour period is known as 16/8 fasting. Alternate-day fasting can help with weight loss and cardiovascular wellbeing on occasion, but 16/8 is the simplest protocol and can be followed nearly every day (with validation from the doctor). For certain individuals, a 16-hour period is the ideal length of time. It won't be as stupid as it looks because you'll be resting for around eight hours out of 16.

1.7 Intermittent Fasting FAQs

Let's answer the most frequently asked questions people have when first starting their intermittent fasting regimen.

1. What are the best times for intermittent fasting?

Intermittent fasting can be done in a number of forms. 16/8, 5:2, 24, and sometimes even 36-hour fasts are among the most common. By far, the most common intermittent fasting plan is 16/8, which was popularized by Martin Berkhan. This fast entails fasting for 16 hours and just feeding over an eight-hour time, as the name implies. This is usually accomplished by enjoying a light dinner and then fasting until the morning.

2. Am I allowed to drink liquids during my fast?

Yes, actually. Zero-calorie drinks such as water, caffeine, and tea are appropriate. Coffee cannot be sweetened. It's possible that small quantities of heavy cream are appropriate. Coffee is especially helpful throughout a fast because it suppresses appetite.

3. How can you transition away from intermittent fasting?

People can move to a 6:1 strategy, according to Michael Mosley, the creator, and promoter of the 5:2 protocol. That is, six days a week, eat a regular diet, and one day a week, try a fasting approach. Others may take a similar approach to the 80 - 20 eating pattern popularized on several exercise and wellness blogs, in which you consume a balanced, healthful diet 80% of the time and engage in more enjoyable meals 20% of the time.

4. Can I work out while fasting?

Fasted exercises are perfectly acceptable. Before a fasted exercise, certain experts suggest getting branched-chain amino acids (BCAAs).

5. How safe is intermittent fasting?

Intermittent fasting may seem to be a cruel or disruptive way of eating, yet as people, we've adapted to it, and it's a style of eating that our bodies are really comfortable with. Yeah, intermittent fasting is safe; nevertheless, it is important to learn when and how to utilize intermittent fasting. It is therefore not recommended for adults who have had an eating problem in the past, pregnant women, breastfeeding mothers, children under the age of 18, or others who are immune damaged. Prior to actually undertaking some lifestyle changes, make sure to check with the doctor first.

6. How Long Do You Follow an IF regimen?

Many people who are considering intermittent fasting have a doubt regarding how long the diet plan would last. Is it possible to sustain an intermittent fasting regimen for an extended period of time? Unfortunately, there is no definitive solution since intermittent fasting is described by no specific eating style; however, researchers have answered that question in studies conducted. Any nutritionists, for example, are concerned with compliance with the diet plan. Fasting days are often exhausting, but ad-libitum feeding is simple to manage.

Furthermore, certain scientists have expressed reservations regarding the efficacy of participating in a long-term regimen involving extreme caloric restriction, claiming that there is insufficient data to tell for certain that it is healthy. Although existing research shows that fasting is unlikely to hurt balanced, normal-weight, unhealthy, or overweight adults emotionally or physically. The lengthy medical benefits of those who follow religious fasting procedures have been studied in several lengthy longitudinal trials. Those that fasted on a regular basis have been less prone to have heart problems or sudden cardiac death in all those reports.

7. Isn't Skipping Breakfast A Bad Idea?

No, it's not true. The issue is that most stereotyped breakfast-skippers lead unhealthy lives. The method is completely safe if you make sure to consume nutritious options for the remainder of the day.

8. May I take supplements during a fast?

Yes, absolutely. Bear in mind, though, that certain supplements, such as fat-soluble vitamins, can function best if consumed with food.

9. Can IF slow down my metabolic rate?

No, it's not true. Brief fasts have been shown in studies to improve metabolic rate. Fasting for three or four days, on the other hand, will slow down the metabolic rate.

10. Is intermittent fasting effective for weight loss?

Intermittent fasting magically and easily reduces body fat. If you do it for a couple of weeks on the spur of the moment, you can see a difference in your body. Of course, getting some physical activity when on a diet is beneficial, particularly if your goal is to drop fat

11. Do I keep track of my calories?

You will avoid the hassle of calorie counting with intermittent fasting. You shouldn't have to count calories except when you're following the 5:2 fasting process. You have two days to count calories and hold it all under 600 kcal for males and 500 kcal for females by using the 5:2 system.

12. Can I eat anything?

While the diet theoretically allows you to consume whatever you want, it is not recommended because it can negatively impact the health. You could have a horrible gas issue if you consume too much fast food when fasting. All kinds of non-nutritious foods should be avoided. Poor diet isn't going to benefit you at all.

13. Wouldn't I be dehydrated if I did IF?

If you ever do not make a deliberate attempt to consume adequate water and liquid during your intermittent fasting time, you are more likely to get dehydrated. You must maintain track of the amount of liquid or fluid you have ingested. Make sure you have at least Eight glasses to meet the mark. It's much healthier if you really can consume upwards of 8 glasses.

14: Should I no longer be concerned with carbohydrates?

Since intermittent fasting allows you to eat anything you like, carbs are also permitted. However, make a deliberate attempt to consume the smallest number of carbohydrates possible every day. Also, prefer complex carbohydrates over refined carbs wherever possible.

15. Who can benefit from intermittent fasting?

IF is beneficial to all. However, men profit from intermittent fasting a little bit more than women. Weight reduction and improved body structure are the main advantages of intermittent fasting. Fasting, on the other hand, has a slew of other nutritional advantages. Enhanced hormone levels, digestive fitness, and insulin sensitivity are only a few of the benefits.

16. Can I stop IF whenever I want?

Fasting does not have a set schedule that you would adhere to for a set amount of time. You can fast whenever you like until you've effectively conditioned your body to abstain from eating when you like. It will take a few weeks for the body to adjust to the new system. So be compliant and cooperative at the time.

Chapter 2: Intermittent Fasting for Women Over 50

In this chapter, all the sections are dedicated to intermittent fasting-related topics in the context of women over 50. We'll start with what the science says about the reasons behind menopause and weight gain in women. We'll also talk about men and women respond differently when it comes to fasting and how IF impacts female hormones for better or worse. Then, a section will highlight the benefits of intermittent fasting for women who have already gone through menopause and wish to lose the resultant weight. In other words, this chapter will give all the information you as an older woman wanting to start intermittent fasting.

2.1 The Science Behind Menopause and Weight Gain

Nearly every single day, you invest hours in the gym as an older woman. Chicken breast, salmon, and vegetables are all you eat. The digits on the scale, on the other hand, refuse to budge — or, maybe, they're steadily rising, alongside your waist size. Menopause is a stressful time in a woman's life. What is it with menopause that causes you to put on weight and makes losing weight even more difficult? It's most likely a combination of menopause and aging-related variables.

Many women experience shifts as a result of the transition, like weight gain that defies all the most determined attempts to remedy it. When it comes to their weight, women often believe that they'll be the root of the issue. Hormonal variations and other changes associated with menopause, though, are often to blame. These have nothing to do with what they're doing.

Recognizing why women gain weight during menopause can assist them in accepting this natural function and knowing how to best monitor their weight in the future to maintain their health. When you reach your mid-to-late 40s as a woman, you may realize that, aside from the irregular flare-up or low mood, your best blue mom jeans are becoming markedly tighter. It isn't in your head this time. According to a classic study, the average female acquires about four and a half lbs. as she enters menopause in her 40s. It's also a pattern that shows no signs of slowing down: According to a new study released in the Mayo Clinic journal, women in their 50s and 60s continue to gain about a pound and a half per year. The primary cause is the natural skeletal muscle that takes place as people get older. Your metabolism slows when muscle burns more calories than fat, allowing you to gain weight. According to science, you lose approximately a half-pound of muscle each year starting at the age of 30, and that amount increases to almost a complete pound by the age of 50.

However, as you progress through menopause, you may recognize different things: Even though the amount on the chart doesn't seem to be rising much, anybody fat you acquire tends to end up amassing all over your stomach, giving you a fat belly. Your ovaries cease releasing estrogen during menopause, and the only area where it can be produced is in your belly fat tissue. As a result, in order to obtain estrogen, the body automatically leans toward fat stores in that area. The stomach has been dubbed "the third ovary" by experts. However, this kind of fat referred to as visceral fat, is hazardous. It develops tension hormones like cortisol and also harmful substances called cytokines. These chemicals cause your body to produce more insulin, which increases fat storage in fat cells while also increasing appetite. As a result, you gain more belly fat ever and are more likely to grow insulin resistance, which is a major risk factor for cardiac failure and type 2 diabetes.

Women's hips and thighs appear to accumulate excess pounds as they're younger, a phenomenon known as gynoid body fat. Hormone fluctuations allow many female bodies to begin accumulating excess weight around the center throughout early menopause than after menopause, a phenomenon known as android fat distribution, which is common in men. Women find it very aggravating. They're not only dealing with hot sweats as well as other hormonal changes issues, but they're also dealing with a significant shift of body shape. It's not just about your looks when you gain weight around your waist. It's a possible health hazard because it's linked to a higher likelihood of medical issues like cardiac disease, stroke, and diabetes. After menopause, this changing extra weight is likely to contribute to women's increased risk of heart disease.

Estrogen's influence Estrogen tends to better regulate body mass in animal research. Lab mice with reduced hormone levels eat too much and are less fit and healthy. Reduced estrogen can often slow the body's metabolic rate, which is the rate at which it transforms accumulated energy into usable energy. Once estrogen levels have dropped since menopause, it's possible that the very same thing affects women. According to some data, estrogen hormone replacement therapy raises a female's basal metabolic rate. This will aid in the slowing of gaining weight. In addition, a loss of estrogen can allow the body to use carbohydrates and sugar levels inefficiently, increasing fat accumulation and making weight loss more difficult.

Other aging considerations play a role as well. Many other modifications occur when women mature, all of which lead to obesity. They're less inclined to workout, for example. Fifteen percent of people are insufficiently active, and this number rises with years of life. Furthermore, as we age, our muscle mass declines, lowering our basal metabolism and rendering it easier to add weight, particularly for women over 50. The pace at which you can expend energy when exercising slows down. If you choose to lose weight by using the same amount of resources as before, you can need to raise the length of time and strength you exercise, regardless of your previous activity levels.

2.2 How Men vs. Women Respond to IF?

Intermittent fasting has a lengthy range of possible advantages, ranging from weight reduction to increased lifespan. Now, a limited yet increasing wealth of studies shows that female's fasts can have unique benefits and disadvantages than male's fasts. Women, in particular, can experience the effects of abstinence faster than men. During fasting, a metabolic mechanism is turned on. When this occurs, you begin to burn fat for energy rather than carbohydrate (or blood glucose). Any of the advantages of some fasting practices may be attributed to this. According to researchers, women can experience the transition faster than men while pursuing an intermittent fasting regimen. When comparing men and women who fasted for equal lengths of time, researchers discovered that women had more fat in their bloodstream. This means that women can benefit from shorter fasting periods. A 16:8 schedule, as opposed to an 18:6 plan, which involves abstinence for 18 hours and eating within a six-hour timeframe, could be more effective for women. Females can profit from significantly smaller fasting timeframes than males, according to animal studies.

Women's fat loss results can be linked to stringent diets as well as fasting. The majority of sporadic fasts don't place any restrictions on anything you should consume during your feeding periods or days. Obese women who fasted intermittently and adopted a strict diet lose more weight, according to a report released in a journal in 2019.

Women's age can also influence how their bodies respond to skipping breakfast. Fasting can cause post-menopausal ladies to lose two times as much fat as youthful, premenopausal ladies, according to experts. According to a report, post-menopausal people shed upwards of 24 lbs. during one year of fasting on alternating days. Post-menopausal ladies lost nine pounds following 90 days of time-restricted diet (also regarded as 16:8).

The truth is that everybody, not just males and females, reacts to fasting differently. In fact, males and females respond to IF in different ways. The gonads react to a hormone named gonadotropin release hormone, which is found in everybody. It induces the ovaries to produce progesterone in women and the testes to generate testosterone in men. Since it is implicated in the menstrual cycle and is dependent on rhythms and patterns, the mechanism is heavily supervised in women. It's likely that improvements in one's behaviors and routines interrupt gonadotropin release hormone more quickly in women than in men, but missing a meal can also create more pain in women than in men. Kisspeptin, a protein that induces increased vulnerability to fasting, was shown to be greater in females. This is only one hypothesis, and further testing is required. However, several rat experiments have shown that fasting has a detrimental impact on female sex hormone, and some human evidence suggests that women have a harder time controlling appetite throughout fasts.

Fasting made men more parasympathetic, implying their stress response was less irritated, while fasting made women more reactive, implying their systems were tenser, more in the "fight - or - flight" mode.

Since you're not creating as much insulin during abstinence, you may become more responsive to its impact (becoming less "insulin resistant"), and since insulin aids food processing and carbohydrate metabolism, many people consider insulin sensitivity to be essential for optimal weight loss. Some literature suggests that alternate-day fasting has distinct implications for women, namely that it negatively influences tolerance to glucose, which is linked to insulin sensitivity, in males but not in males.

One research found that while men fast for brief amounts of time, their metabolic rate improves by up to 14 percent. Furthermore, according to another analysis, the male body increases testosterone use and human growth hormone development. All of these biochemical modifications are essential for tight muscles and a lower risk of disease. Women, on the other hand, do not react

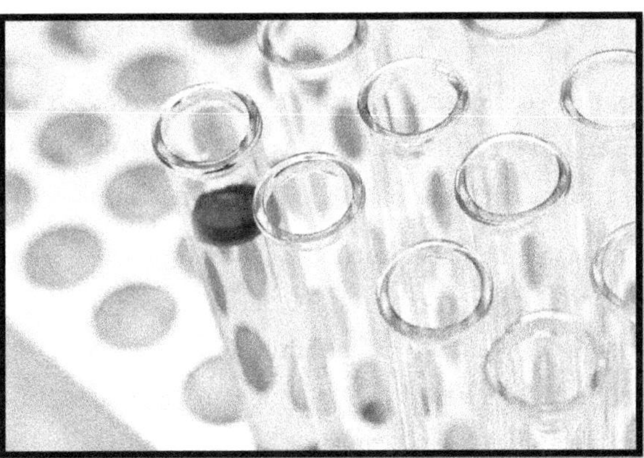

to intermittent fasting in the same way as men do. Another research discovered that while IF increased insulin response in male participants, it had little effect on female subjects. In reality, the tolerance to sugar in women deteriorated. Other studies on the impact of IF on blood lipids showed that men's "healthy" cholesterol remained unchanged while their lipids declined, whereas women's "good" cholesterol increased while their lipids held steady.

2.3 How IF Affects Female Hormones?

Tinkering with intermittent fasting can appear insignificant in the big scheme of things when it comes to health decisions. Well, it's a greater issue for certain women than you would think. It turns out that the hormones that control important functions like ovulation, digestion, and even mood are highly responsive to caloric intake. In reality, modifying your eating habits, like how often and what you consume, may have a detrimental effect on your sex hormone.

The hypothalamic-pituitary-gonadal axis is one mechanism by which fasting impacts reproductive hormones in both males and females. Luckily, the HPG axis is the more general name for this. It's not necessary to understand how the HPG axis functions, but if you're curious, here's what ends up happening: GnRH (gonadotropin-releasing hormone) is released by the hypothalamus in frequent bursts known as "pulses." The pituitary gland responds to GnRH pulses by releasing luteinizing hormone (LH) and follicle-stimulating hormone (FSH) (FSH). The gonads are then affected by LH and FSH.

LH and FSH promote the development of estrogen and progesterone in women, which are needed for the release of eggs (ovulation) and the maintenance of a pregnancy. They increase androgens and sperm output in males. Since this sequence of interactions occurs in women on a very particular, daily basis, GnRH bursts must be precisely coordinated. Otherwise, anything will go awry. Periods come to an end when no eggs are produced. Fasting can set off GnRH pulses, which appear to be very responsive to external stimuli. Even a three-day fast will cause these hormone rhythms to change in certain women. There's also proof that skipping a full meal isn't a disaster in and of itself, but it still can set off our biochemical system's alarm.

For a long time, scientists thought that a woman's body fat proportion controlled her reproductive capacity. The premise is that if your body's fat fell below a percentage—roughly 11%—hormones would just get totally messed up, and your monthly cycle would end. So, if you're dropping fat mass, your system might think there's not anything to eat and attempt and stop you from reproducing. However, the matter is more complex than that. And before fat mass levels decrease, women's bodies are on high alert. Women that aren't very slim can even eliminate menstruating and miss their cycles as a consequence. That's why the total energy equation—how much calories you consume versus how much you "expend"—might be more critical than body fat in this phase.

When it comes to abstinence or severely calorie restriction, males and females seem to react differently. Kisspeptin, a protein-like chemical important in the reproductive phase, may be to blame. Kisspeptin activates the development of GnRH in both genders, and we know it's responsive to hormones like insulin, leptin, and ghrelin, which control and respond to hunger and satiety. Kisspeptin levels are higher in females than in males. Women's bodies could be more vulnerable to shifts in energy expenditure if they have more Kisspeptin. Fasting allows women's Kisspeptin output to drop more quickly than men's. As Kisspeptin levels fall, GnRH levels fall out of whack, disrupting the entire monthly hormone cycle.

Females, who fast, on the other hand, seem to consume much less protein since they are consuming less altogether. This is a challenge since protein contains essential nutrients, which are essential for reproduction. If you don't get enough amino acids, it may trigger the estrogen receptors as well as a hormone named insulin-like growth factor (IGF-1). And during the monthly period, both are used to plump up the uterine lining. If the uterine lining does not firm up, an egg would not be able to penetrate, and reproduction would not be possible.

Estrogen has a major impact on a woman's appetite, temperament, reproduction, and body mass index. Estrogen serves more than just the prostate and fertility. Estrogen sensors can be found in the brains, Digestive system passages, and bones, among other places. When hormone levels fluctuate, biochemical functions such as cognition, temperament, metabolism, regeneration, protein turnover, bone structure, and, perhaps most importantly, food intake and energy equilibrium are all affected. Estrogens alter the peptides that tell you whether you're complete (cholecystokinin) or starving (ghrelin) in the brainstem (ghrelin). Estrogens also activate neurons in the hypothalamus, which stop the development of appetite-regulating proteins. If you're someone who allows your hormone levels to drop quickly, you may notice yourself getting a lot hungrier and consuming a ton more than you might under normal conditions.

It's possible that women's bodies are more sensitive to shifts in energy expenditure. When their systems sense differences, the HPG-axis can be disrupted, throwing the entire hormone cycle off. Fasting will lower hormone levels, which can lead to a rise in hunger and lipid accumulation. Women who are concerned with controlling their weight after menopause have higher amounts of cortisol, a stress response, than women who are not. When you add on the poor sleep that comes with menopause, the "tension tank" is quickly filling up. Reduced hormone levels also indicate a reduced body's ability to cope with stress. The bucket is filling up a lot faster than it used to be. Even though certain stressors are beneficial to our health, such as workouts, studying, and progress, we will only become healthier if we allow ourselves to rebound from them. So, if you're a woman going through this hormonal change, just consider intermittent fasting if: Your stress level is small.

- You're having a good night's sleep every single night.

- Hot flashes and mood fluctuations (luckily) don't plague you.

- There are no nutrient deficiencies in your body.

- You are not terribly stressed.

2.4 Post-Menopausal Benefits of Intermittent Fasting

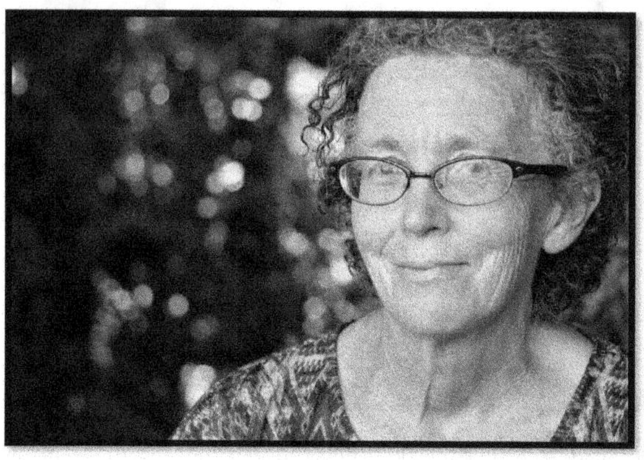

Intermittent fasting is beneficial to women of all ages, from their early twenties into early menopause, menopause, and through their older years. When it comes to the effects of intermittent fasting, there is emerging research and data that suggest a distinct effect on women and men. One of the main causes behind this disparity being because female bodies are more suited to retaining fat and are drastically altered once fasting starts. Fasting with a low or zero-calorie consumption may have negative consequences for certain people, like cramps and shifts in the menstrual cycle. This can happen after a long time of abstinence, though for both males and females, the majority of the adverse effects or pain involved with not eating is just temporary.

IF has many benefits for women over 50, all of which are linked to hormone levels and their development. Women with high insulin sensitivity have more stable blood glucose levels. In just a few weeks of fasting, something happens. This appears to be stable over time, with average increases in insulin remaining at usual amounts.

Women lose more bone density than males when they become older. Lean mass preservation is critical at all periods of life, but especially so when people get older. The conservation of lean muscle is higher as calories are limited by fasting instead of food constrained regimes that do not contain fasts. This assists in weight management by assisting the body in breaking down fat.

Many individuals are affected by depression, which may lead to other behaviors like bingeing and not having enough exercise. One analysis found that after two months of intermittent fasting, depressive symptoms dropped significantly. This involves a large number of people at various points of their lives, including postpartum, perimenopause, and menstrual cycles. While fasting is not recommended throughout pregnancy or breastfeeding, consuming regular, balanced meals can provide you with anything you need before you are prepared to start an IF process.

Inflammation is minimized, and inflammation and excess weight linked to chronic diseases demonstrate significant improvement over time. Since persistent inflammation may lead to obesity, this may lead to weight management as well as weight loss. Similarly, fasting is very important in terms of post-menopausal women's health because tummy fat is linked to a greater incidence of heart disease and stroke in post-menopausal females than males. This fat can produce chronic inflammation and other molecules, which may raise the risk of a heart attack, liver damage, hypertension, and other illnesses.

Women over the age of 50 can experience enhanced heart rewards. Intermittent fasting resulted in a 20% reduction in the low-density lipoprotein (LDL) cholesterol, a 20% decline in hypertension, and a 20% to 40% significant decrease in metabolic syndrome in post-menopausal people. Low LDL cholesterol levels and blood pressure raise the risk of heart failure and stroke, while insulin tolerance opens the way for diabetes. These enhancements can aid in the prevention of diabetes and heart disease.

Bone health protection is another advantage of IF for older women. According to a report reported in 2017 in Healthy Aging, skipping breakfast does not trigger bone deterioration in the same manner as daily dieting does. The dramatic drop in estrogen levels that occurs after menopause will impair bone strength, raising the likelihood of the fragile bone condition osteoporosis. This is significant because women account for 75 percent of the approximate 10 million Individuals who have osteoporosis. There is research connecting cycles of fasting to better bone health, as studies suggest that fasting affects the way female bodies manufacture hormones that influence bone minerals, including phosphate and calcium.

As per a report, abstinence for various periods of time reduced the incidence of severe diseases in older people, with most of the literature focusing on the benefits of fasting on cancer. Fasting does seem to block some of the mechanisms that contribute to cancers and may also delay tumor development, according to the report. Many results indicate that women who follow various fasting strategies saw improvements in their moods and self-esteem, as well as a decline in anxiety and depression, according to studies.

2.5 Is Intermittent Fasting Safe for Older Women?

So, is IF safe for older women or just women in general? It all actually depends on your health goals and current health status. Some scientists say that skipping breakfast can cause hormone levels disruptions, which can give rise to mood changes and fertility issues; whereas others assert that it's completely fine so long as people listen to the body and follow the directions. So, what's the big deal? Let's look at whether females should fast intermittently and, if so, how to do it and safely.

According to experts, it all narrows back to your general stress tolerance. Women's brains work in the opposite way than men's. They're programmed in such a way that chronic stress to the body can disrupt a female's hormone levels processes. Although the word "stress" has a negative meaning, it is not all awful. Many wellness practices, such as strength training and the paleo diet, put your body under stress. Such activities enhance profound, healthy effects on the body if you manage your load well. Even so, if you're already stressed out, your body might not be capable of handling anymore. Fasting, which doctors describe as a "hermetic stressor," can create bad hormonal changes rather than the planned health effects in this case.

Remember that you should only last for 12 to 16 hours at a time, not for days. You also have plenty of food to relax and savor a delicious and healthy meal. After all, a few other older ladies may require frequent eating associated with metabolic syndromes or medication instructions. In that scenario, you must talk to your doctor about your daily diet before taking any action.

While it isn't theoretically fasting, some physicians claim that allowing incredibly simple foods like whole fruit mostly during the fasting frame has health benefits. Adjustments such as these can still provide a much-needed break for your intestinal and metabolic systems. For instance, the famous weight-loss book "Fit for Life" recommended consuming just fruit after dinner and then before noon.

In fact, according to the authors of this book, they had individuals who really only altered their food patterns by fasting for 12 to 16 hours each day. Despite not adhering to this diet's other guidelines or counting calories, they lost all that weight and improved their health. This method may have worked simply because dieters swapped sugary snacks for whole food products. In any case, participants found this change in diet to be straightforward and easier to implement. Purists won't call this fasting, but it's critical to note that you have alternatives if you can't go without food for more than a few hours.

Excess weight, metabolic syndrome, and other related signs of menopause can all be managed with intermittent fasting. Intermittent fasting, however, causes mild stress to the body, so if you do have chronic fatigue or a serious disease, you may want to avoid incorporating it into your normal schedule. Give heed to how you feel if you decide to try intermittent fasting. If skipping breakfast means you feel too anxious, or if you become weak or ill while fasting, you should either cut your fast short or stop fasting altogether. It's also worth noting that you shouldn't have to fast each day. You can fast once a week or just a handful of days a week if you want to.

Menopause can be a tricky process, but with the appropriate diet and exercise, you can stay in shape, thrilled, and comfortable as your hormones fluctuate. For more information to help you live a healthier life, get yourself acquainted with common menopause myths and blood glucose stability during menopause. In any particular instance, it also seems that IF works best for elderly ladies as it's relatively simple to follow. By lessening consumption windows, they claim it tends to help them generally restrict calorie intake and make healthier food choices. According to some studies, IF leads to enhanced weight burning while protecting lean body mass, making it a better

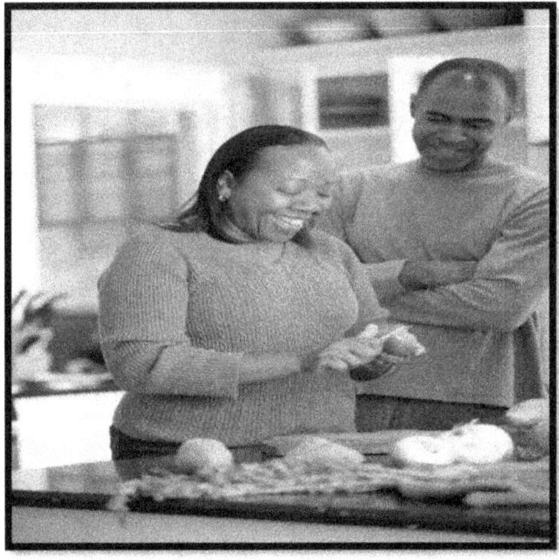

option than simply reducing calories, refined sugars, or fat. Of course, the majority of people combine IF with yet another weight-loss strategy. To lose weight, you could perhaps try and eat 1,200 kcal intake per day. It may well be important to distribute out 1,200 kcal over two main meals and two snacks rather than three meals and three snacks.

The fact of the matter is that each and every female is unique. Some women thrive on fasting, while others are more receptive to the physical stress it causes. While there is a huge amount of evidence from older ladies who have actually experienced benefits from decreased hunger pangs to good sleep to elevated mood, there's not enough scholarly data to make firm conclusions just yet.

2.6 Helpful Tips for Older Women Starting IF

Exercise and nutritious food become essential than before during early menopause and post-menopause. Sustaining lean mass and avoiding excess weight should be a top priority. Please remember that just because the rest of humanity seems to be doing it, this might not be the best option for you. The "hangry" mode is real, and it can be incredibly intolerable if you're dealing with a lot of pressure so, if you're still interested in doing IF, there's a proper way to go about it. Here are some suggestions for women over 50 who are new to IF or women in general.

1. Begin with Physical Activity

Exercise can help to reduce the adverse effects of estrogen deficit. While hormone treatment can help reduce body composition and abdominal obesity, it has no effect on basal energy output, which means it won't help you substantially increase the number of calories at rest as more musculature can. According to research, post-menopausal females who participate in a thorough fitness routine benefit from living a healthy lifestyle, high bone density, and psychological wellbeing. It's never too late to get into shape. Start gradually and concentrate on your aspirations. Walking on a regular basis can help with Vitamin D absorption and overall health. Simply move at a rapid pace to get your heart racing. Begin with a group session or have an instructor show you the moves if you've never been to a gym before. It is understandable how challenging it can be.

2. Concentrate on Nutrition

Your greatest weapon is to eat well. You don't have to skip breakfast or keep track of every single bite. To begin, make sure you're getting sufficient protein. Intend for 30grams of protein per meal. It's also critical to consume a diverse range of nutrients in order to protect our bone fragments and tissues. Fruit and veg obviously, are included. Fatty fish, such as tuna and salmon, are high in Omega-3 and omega-6 fatty acids, which have been associated with better mental state and cardiovascular health. If you dislike salmon as many people do, you might want to consider taking a fish oil pill. Most importantly, don't put too much restriction on your diet. A reasonable caloric deficit of 250–300 kcal per day is ideal. According to healthcare professionals, extreme limitation triggers the famous malnourishment reaction. Your brain reacts by increasing your appetite, making high-fat corn syrup food products difficult to resist.

3. Just Go Slow

Fasting may be beneficial to women of all ages and stages, and you might realize that you enjoy it. You should still begin progressively to see how the body reacts with smaller and kinder periods of fasting a couple of days a week. You might find that abstinence isn't for you, and that's perfectly fine! Discover a groove that brings you joy. That is the most critical thing. Instead of a strict regular fast, pick 2 or 3 different days per week (for instance, Tuesday, Thursday, and Saturdays) and attempt a smaller fast on all those days; 12-14 hours is a reasonable way to consider. You'll also reap all of the effects of fasting, but the hormones won't be as shocked as they would be if you fasted every day. If you like performing brief fasts only a few days a week, you can still lengthen them or introduce a few more days to see just how you cope.

Doing everything in one go is always a recipe for disaster. Assume you've selected the 16:8 strategy. You make the decision to begin the next day. If you always had breakfast at 8 a.m., there's no reason to force yourself to wait before noon on the first day. It's fine if you have to make a transition but do it very slowly. Breakfast could be postponed for 1 hour, then maybe 2 hours, and so forth. It takes a few weeks to be comfortable skipping breakfast. Migraines, lightheadedness, low appetite and overall frustration over not eating will all be avoided by gradually growing the fasting window.

4. Be Flexible about it

One of the advantages of IF is that it allows you to consume foods that you would have previously limited (for example, carbs or pizza). It enables you to consume bigger meals. So, when you're limiting your feeding time, don't limit yourself too much in terms of what you consume. To put it another way, don't consume a little side salad day after day. Eat whatever you want, as long as it's within justification. After dinner, get a large plate of food and a treat — and a few sips of champagne! You want to be sure you're consuming plenty during your consuming time that you won't be starving throughout the abstinence window the next day. Aim for 80 to 90 percent of the time to eat healthier, including meat, complex carbs, and good fats.

5. Drink a lot of water

Try to drink 12 ounces of water within one hour of waking up. Consume about 12 ounces or upwards if you start to feel hungry. Fasting has shown that what you initially keep mistaking for hunger is very likely boredom or fatigue. Drinking plenty of water during the day can keep your appetite satisfied, leave you feeling more alert, and satisfy the urge or habit to eat something. Keep away from zero-calorie energy beverages and chemical sweeteners, and just enjoy coffee, hot tea, or sparkling water.

If you like the book don't forget to leave me a review on Amazon.

It's important to me! Thank you.

Martha Kirby

Chapter 3: A Guide to Intermittent Fasting and Food

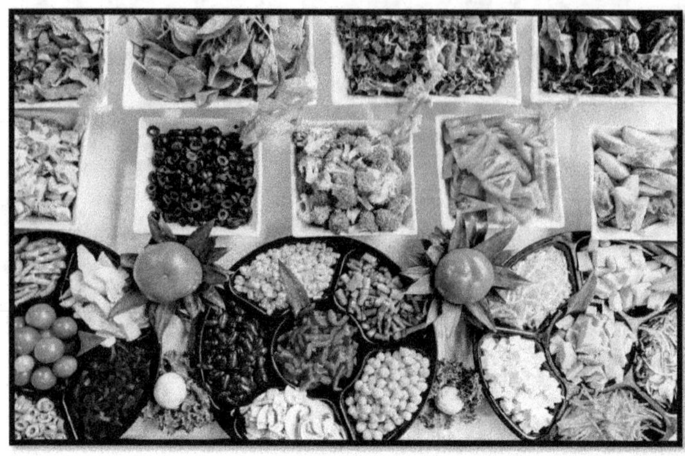

In this chapter, we'll talk about everything related to intermittent fasting and food. The sections will be dedicated to the best and worst foods to eat on an IF eating plan, along with the best foods to break your fast with.

3.1 What To Eat And Avoid On IF Diet?

IF is gaining momentum; perhaps the attraction arises from the absence of dietary restrictions. When you can eat is regulated, but what you can eat is not. That being said, what you consume too is relevant. Will you be breaking your fast with bottles of wine, frozen yogurt, and packages of cheese slices? Very likely not. So, let's have a peek at the best foods to incorporate into your IF diet.

1. Healthy Grains

Carbs are a necessary aspect of life and are not the villain when it comes to losing weight. Since you'll be fasting for a significant portion of the day during this plan, it's vital to plan time for how you'll get enough calories without feeling bloated. While a balanced diet excludes refined foods, there is a place or time for the whole-wheat, breakfast sandwiches, and bread rolls, which absorb more easily and provide fast and simple energy. These can be a perfect supply of fuel when out and about if you want to your daily workouts or practice daily during intermittent fasting.

2. Papaya

You'll probably start to feel hungry in the final moments of your fast, particularly if you're new to skipping meals. This can lead to you overeating in large amounts, making you exhausted and groggy moments later. Papain, a special enzyme present in papaya, works on amino acids to break them down. Incorporating pieces of this sweet fruit into a high-protein meal will aid absorption and reduce bloating.

3. Water

Being hydrated is important on any diet, but especially on an intermittent fasting diet. It is important not to get drained when fasting. Per day, you must consume at least eight cups of liquid. Make it a habit to drink the water each half an hour. You should also fill a 1-liter water bottle with water and leave it somewhere visible so that any time you glance at it, you are reminded to stay hydrated. Many women experience pregnancy complications as a result of excessive water use. However, if you do not consume sufficient water, your fitness will deteriorate, and your digestive complications will worsen. Dehydration induces a slew of other concerns in the body, including jaundice, exhaustion, headaches, and dizziness.

If you can't drink water, consider fruit drinks, raw vegetables, coconut water, and other related liquids. Fruit shakes are also another choice, but they contain so many calories that one glass should suffice for the entire day. If you're using the 5:2 form of extended fasting, avoiding the smoothie is a smart choice because it's definitely high in calories.

4. Legumes and Beans

Although many diets ignore legumes and beans completely due to their high carbohydrate content, skipping breakfast allows you to periodically indulge in a tub of legume and bean-packed chili. Beans and grains are super useful to your well-being. They are low in calories and leave you content for a lot longer. A balanced diet can have a variety of foods, and legumes are one of them. You should eat grains and beans a minimum of three days a week, if not more. It will also assist you in losing weight and establishing a healthy eating schedule. Consuming fast food is often significantly worse than consuming calorie-dense real foods. Beans and legumes may be used in a range of dishes. While Cuban chili can come to mind first, grains and beans may be used in a variety of other dishes, including curries, stews, sauces, and even roasting. Try frying chickpeas, lentils, or peas with pepper and salt if you're searching for lunch. In less than 10 minutes, you'll have a great tasting snack with no chemical flavors.

5. Potatoes

Unlike most diets, fasting has few carb limits or constraints. So, if potatoes are your thing, you're in fortune. According to health specialists, consuming potatoes throughout fasting is beneficial. Potatoes are the greatest comfort food in every country, and because of their high value, they can be found all year long. It is also moderately priced. It's often regarded as among the most filling items. White potatoes are easily digested by the human body. They're still a decent exercise snack when mixed with a source of protein to refresh the tired and hungry body. Another advantage of potatoes for the IF diet plan is that when they are cooled, they turn into complex carbohydrate that fuels healthy bacteria in the digestive tract.

6. Avocado

Avocado is one of those fruits that deserve to be listed on its own to highlight its importance! One avocado can sustain you working for at least 6 hours. There would be no hungry bouts or lightheadedness afterward. It's chock-full of all the positive stuff. It is, of course, one of the higher calorie foods, so you may question whether you should consume it as part of a weight-loss diet. However, a study has shown that it offers decent protein, which really is essential for fat-burning. It helps you stay satisfied for a long time, but you don't consume other fast food or indulge for a prolonged period of time. This way, you're not eating too much, which helps you lose weight. When the avocado is fully mature, it may be consumed on its own. You can create a feta cheese and avocado bowl with it, as well as guacamole, avocado smoothies, and tasty dips.

7. Egg

The egg is a nutrient-dense meal. The neurons need a certain amount of fat, which is present in eggs. An egg may be used in a variety of ways, including breakfast, lunch, and dinner in the shape of egg curry. Eggs are necessary for baked goods, and if you like baking, using eggs in your standard meals is not a challenge. It will maintain you pumped up for at least 4 hours. Fasting may be taxing on the brain and mind, but getting superfood like an egg on hand is definitely a safe idea.

8. Berries

Flavonoids are abundant in berries. They have a magical impact on health and hair. You will see how berries are often used in skincare items and advertisements. It is done purposefully: berries help to maintain the skin smooth and fresh. Berries such as blueberry, cherry, mulberry, mango, among others, are all helpful to one's well-being. They're also delicious. You don't have to think about calories if you consume half a cup of just about any berry a day. Berries also are tasty, but they can be consumed on their own. However, you can use them in savory dishes as well as pies, cookies, milkshakes, and juices. Cooked strawberries work as well.

9. Chicken

As previously mentioned, skipping breakfast does not preclude all foods, and poultry is one which anyone likes but also can handle adequately whilst on a diet. Tiny amounts of poultry can be used in your standard menu if you observe fasting. White meat is already thought to be beneficial to one's welfare. It does not trigger any of the health issues that processed meat may. In every region of the country, poultry and duck are easily available. Since turkey bird is not bred all over the world, you will need to do some research. Different forms of birds may also be served with a minimal serving amount. It's critical to monitor your meals whether you want to lose fat or enjoy a healthy lifestyle.

Foods to Avoid on Intermittent Fasting

Beginners sometimes make the error of consuming just about everything throughout their whole eating periods. They mistakenly think that all calorie intakes are equivalent and that the organs can burn the food they consume over the next abstinence period. Although your body will burn food, particularly fat, throughout your fast, you must always watch your diet for maximum performance.

The following foods must be stopped at all costs, but particularly during fasting diet feeding windows, when what you consume at that period has a direct effect on your body and well-being.

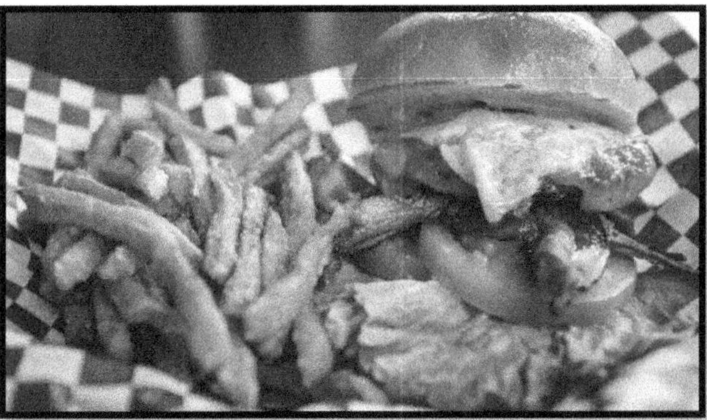

These foods can be avoided since they are high in calories and contain a lot of starch, fat, and salt. They won't satisfy you after a short, and they might even leave you hungry. They often have so little nutrition.

1. Saturated and Trans Fats

Deep-fried products, artificial butter, and other butter substitutes, processed baked products; popcorn, candies, and a variety of other ready meals all contain trans-fats. This kind of fat is very unhealthy because it raises bad cholesterol, causes inflammation, and increases the risk of cardiovascular failure. Some foods, oils, and dairy goods include saturated fats. They are suitable in balance and are a strong choice for ketogenic diets and fasting. Although they cannot be eliminated, they should be consumed in moderation with optimal performance.

2. Preservatives and Sugary Foods

Fruit sugars are antioxidants that are good for you that have no negative effects on your body. Refined sugars can be removed in sauces, desserts, frozen treats, candies, and other items. Monk fruit and xylitol are two sugar replacements that will please your sweet tooth while holding your blood glucose in control. Both are made from plant sources that do not involve sugar. Limit the following foods if you choose to stick to an intermittent diet plan:

- Sugar

- Barbecue sauce

- Fruit juice

- Cakes

- Ketchup

- Cereals

- Biscuits

- Popcorn heated in the microwave

- Sugary granola

- Potato chips

3. Excessive Amounts of Carb-Filled Foods

In limited to medium amounts, grains (buckwheat, rice, barley, wheat, and so on) may be a component of a balanced lifestyle. They have sustained energy and can be consumed before a long-distance athletic exercise, such as a sprint or riding, as a power source. Add rolled oats, sesame seeds, and other related seeds and nuts to reduce grains in Greek yogurt or cereal.

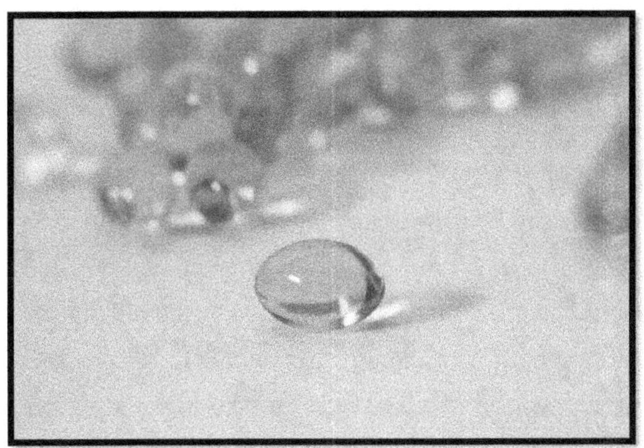

3.2 Best Supplements for Intermittent Fasting

Despite the numerous possible advantages of fasting, it does have one drawback: nutrient loss. Fasting causes your body to lack the nutrition it normally gets from food, particularly if you exercise. The only way to compensate for this lack of nutrition is to consume high-nutrient meals at mealtime. Some individuals, though, do not get many nutrients and vitamins from eating. Supplements may help fasters fill nutrient shortages in this situation. Individuals who fast (or follow a time-restricted diet) on a daily basis will benefit from these supplements in particular.

1. Vitamin D

Vitamin D deficiency is a normal occurrence. Fortunately, a quick blood examination will tell you whether you lack this immunity-increasing vitamin. Doctors still advise that you continue to reach your requirements by getting the sunlight every day. Some individuals, however, can need supplementation. Take the vitamin D with food in these situations because it is fat-soluble that indicates the body requires fat to consume it properly.

2. Branch Chain Amino Acid (BCAA)

BCAAs (branched-chain amino acids) are a class of protein (valine, isoleucine, and leucine). We can't create important proteins on our own, so we need to get them from food. They're contained in important foods like poultry, beef, and dairy. Although this muscle-building supplement is best for those who love fasted cardio or intense exercises first thing in the morning, it may also be eaten during the day (fasting or not) to save the body from being catabolic and preserving lean muscle mass. BCAAs help to protect musculature from disintegrating by encouraging our bodies to utilize energy from food for longer periods of time, making them a strong substitute for skipping breakfast. Another benefit of BCAAs is that they tend to relieve muscle pain after an exercise.

3. Calcium

A regular calcium consumption of 1,000 mg is suggested for adults, which is approximately equal to 3 cups of milk. With a smaller eating time, chances to consume this much can be restricted, so high-calcium products should be prioritized. Vitamin D enhanced milk improves calcium intake and helps to maintain bone strength. You should add the milk to beverages or cereals, or simply consume it with meals, to increase your regular calcium intake. Non-dairy calcium options contain tofu and soy goods and also green vegetables like kale if you're not a lover of the shakes.

4. Collagen

One of the essential components of chicken soup is collagen. It may be obtained in fine powder and incorporated into milkshakes or other liquids to further promote the development of soft tissues, lungs, tendons, and muscles. Collagen starts to break down into an easier form to digest and enhance certain body components when ingested. Collagen, like intermittent fasting, tends to increase muscle strength and helps to reduce bone loss. It's also good for the heart, brain, cognition, metabolism, and losing weight.

5. Multivitamins

One plausible explanation for why intermittent fasting causes fat loss is that the body will have less time to consume and thus consumes fewer calories. Although the idea of fuel in and fuel out stands true, the possibility of vitamin deficiency while in a calorie deficit is seldom addressed. While a multivitamin isn't needed if you eat a well-balanced diet rich in fruits and veggies, living can get intense, and supplementation can really fill the gaps.

6. MCT oil (Medium Chain Triglycerides)

Coconut oil is used to produce MCT oil, which is a form of fat. It has almost no flavor and maybe mixed with coffee or other beverages or consumed by spoonfuls. It can be seen in bulletproof coffee every day. It encourages brain development and movement, thus providing a safe fat-burning energy supply. During their fast, some people drink coffee that contains MCT oil, clarified butter, cocoa butter, or ghee. Oil can weaken a fast, but it will not break ketosis, so it will hold you satiated before your next meal.

3.3 Best Foods to Break Your Fast

Breaking your fast should be easy. So here are some of the best foods to help you break your intermittent or even prolonged fast.

1. Apple Cider Vinegar

Apple Cider Vinegar is a kind of vinegar made from apples. Seven thousand years earlier, apple cider vinegar was being used for its medicinal advantages. Breaking a fast with apple cider vinegar is one of the finest things you can do. It r Reduces the possibility of overeating by increasing satiety. According to studies, it also helps you lose weight by lowering blood sugar levels, improving insulin sensitivity, and stimulating fat burning. ACV frequently produces mitigating chemicals and ions in the liver and intestine. In addition, apple cider vinegar aids digestion in a variety of forms. Apple cider vinegar, for example, can assist with gastrointestinal acidity, gall bladder activity, and fat metabolism. As a result, it aids those who have difficulty absorbing fats in breaking their fast. It also helps people who are unable to generate sufficient digestive enzymes. As a result, using apple cider to break a fast may be beneficial. Furthermore, vinegar makes it easier for fasting newcomers to introduce healthier fats into the diet.

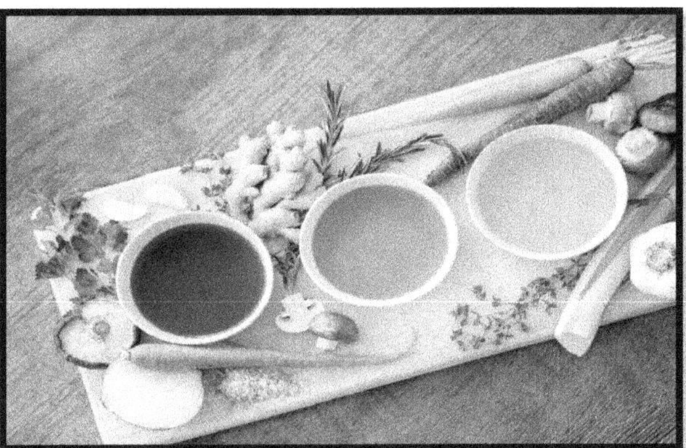

Until you break your fast, take some ACV. This way, you'll get two extra perks before the next meal. It can activate the intestinal tract, aid absorption, and help you feel satisfied after your first meal. Even if you don't eat a lot while attempting to break a fast, it's a surefire way to prevent bingeing.

2. Fish

Fish is a decent source of protein that you should eat while you're breaking your fast or as your first steady meal afterward. If you want to be careful when stopping the fast, start with a bowl of fish stew before moving on to fish meat. Fish, on the other side, may not be an issue for the first meal since it would not place too much pressure on most people's digestive tracts. Additionally, fish, including salmon and mackerel, provide the below nutrition:

- Omega-3 fatty acids (DHA and EPA)

- Vitamin B and D

- Calcium

- Potassium

- Selenium

- Niacin (vitamin B3)

3. Bone Broth

Bone broth includes a ton of electrolytes, so it's great for after a fast. Since mineral degradation is one of the biggest problems when fasting, bone broths include potassium, calcium, magnesium, and sodium. After the quick has cleansed the stomach, consuming bone broth can aid in the absorption of vitamins and minerals from the soup and the meal you'll consume afterward. Bone broth could be the right food to end a fast because fasting causes the body to lose fluids and electrolytes by draining glucose stocks. Also, it tastes amazing thanks to the organic fatty acids.

Sodium, calcium, magnesium, and potassium are all basic electrolytes found in bone broth; following a fast broth aids in the absorption of nutrients from both the broth and other meals. Bone broth may also include collagen for hair, skin, organs, and muscles, as well as enhance sleep by containing necessary amino acids, including glycine, as well as regulate blood sugar and improve the immune system. It also soothes the stomach and provides healthier good fats without the use of carbs.

4. Chicken

Among the most common sources of protein is often one of the healthiest options for breaking a fast. As a result, it's no surprise that poultry is readily digestible for the majority of people. As a consequence, poultry is the most tried and tested meat for breaking a fast. You may also use it to make chicken broth, which is great for ending long fasts. You should pass on to the poultry after your gut has cooled down after drinking some broth. Often eat with the skin while ending the fast since the collagen that protects skin, hair, tissues, and joints is stored there. Chicken also includes essential nutrients such as:

- Magnesium

- Potassium

- Selenium

- B Vitamins

- Niacin (vitamin B3)

5. Butter and Ghee from Grass-Fed Cows

Because good fats are crucial for digestive health, grass-fed fat and ghee should also be included among the best foods for breaking a fast. Butter is really the only milk food that can be used to end a fast safely since it includes little or no lactose. Since ghee is devoid of milk proteins, clarified butter is a safer option. The distinction between the two products is appropriate eating with plants and grasses.

Butyrates, or butyric acid esters, are healthy short-chain fats that fuel the gut microbes, assisting in the maintenance of gastrointestinal equilibrium. Grass-fed milk often has around six times the amount of linoleic acid as grain-fed milk. Although this particular fatty acid assists in the removal of body weight, it also aids in the maintenance of muscle strength, which is helpful to the fasting goals. Grass-fed butter and ghee are rich in nutrients like:

- Vitamin A

- Vitamin K2

- Beta-carotene

- Omega-3 fatty acids

Chapter 4: Get Started With Intermittent Fasting

This chapter will contain all the details of when to start and break your Fasting and consuming periods. A 4-week action plan will be presented to you here. The first week will start from 16:8, and the fasting window will then grow incrementally every week. For each day, sample snacks and meals are presented just to give you an idea of the number of nutrients that are to be consumed so that you don't go below that even if you're not feeling hungry. Furthermore, each day also has an exercise suggestion for you to follow to speed up your weight loss results. For the fasting periods, suggestions are presented for when you might want to have some tea, coffee, or bone broth, as these beverages are allowed during the fasting window and can be consumed at any time during the fasting window.

4.1 Your 4-week Intermittent Fasting Plan

Week 1: 16:8 Fasting

Your first week when first starting your IF journey will have the 16:8 schedule. You will start your eating window from 6:00 am and end it at 2:00 pm. Therefore, your breakfast would be as early as 6:00 am, and your last meal will be your lunch at around 2:00 pm. This schedule will allow you to have a big meal at the start of your day, i.e., your breakfast followed by a mid-morning snack and, finally, lunch. If you wake up on time and have your breakfast at 6:00 am sharp, you can also shift your lunch food to 11:00 am, and therefore have the mid-morning snack between 1:00 pm and 2:00 pm right before your fasting window starts. It's all up to you as to what suits your liking best.

(Week 1 - Part I)

Day 1: (6 am to 2 pm)

Day	Time	Fasting/eating	Exercise
Monday	12 am	Fasting (sleeping)	
	2 am	Fasting (sleeping)	
	4 am	Fasting (sleeping)	

Day	Time	Fasting/eating	Exercise
	6 am	Breakfast: Tea or Coffee Homemade pancakes with fresh fruit and whipped cream	
	8 am		
	10 am		
	12 pm	Lunch: Lasagna (between 12 - 2 pm)	
	2 pm	Fasting	
	4 pm	Fasting	
	6 pm	Fasting	
	8 pm	Fasting	
	10 pm	Fasting (sleeping)	
	12 am	Fasting (sleeping)	

Day 2: (6 am to 2 pm)

Day	Time	Fasting/eating	Exercise
Tuesday	12 am	Fasting (sleeping)	

	2 am	Fasting (sleeping)	
	4 am	Fasting (sleeping)	
	6 am	Breakfast: Tea or Coffee Fried eggs, bacon and sweet potato hash browns	
	8 am		Cycling (1 hour)
	10 am	Snack: carrots sticks	
	12 pm	Lunch: Anti-pesto plate: olives, cheese, cucumbers, fish (if you like), cherry tomatoes, etc.(between 12 - 2 pm)	
	2 pm	Fasting	
	4 pm	Fasting	
	6 pm	Fasting	
	8 pm	Fasting	
	10 pm	Fasting (sleeping)	
	12 am	Fasting (sleeping)	

Day 3: (6 am to 2 pm)

Day	Time	Fasting/eating	Exercise
Wednesday	12 am	Fasting (sleeping)	
	2 am	Fasting (sleeping)	
	4 am	Fasting (sleeping)	
	6 am	Breakfast: Tea or Coffee Crepes with fresh fruit, cinnamon and/or maple syrup	Jog for 30-60 minutes
	8 am	Work	
	10 am	Snack: Raw vegetables (celery, carrots)	
	12 pm	Lunch: Tuna sandwich or tuna salad with pickles (between 12 - 2 pm)	
	2 pm	Fasting	
	4 pm	Fasting	
	6 pm	Fasting	Dance/aerobics class or any low-impact cardio and weights

	8 pm	Fasting	
	10 pm	Fasting (sleeping)	
	12 am	Fasting (sleeping)	

(Week 1 - Part II)

In the second part of week 1, your fasting window will end in the afternoon, and the eating window will range from 12:00 pm to 8:00 pm. You can adjust the timing of your meals anywhere within those 8 hours as you see fit. Even though snacks are not presented in the tables, you can still have at least a snack in the time between your lunch and dinner, if you like it that way.

Day 4: (12 pm to 8 pm)

Day	Time	Fasting/eating	Exercise
Thursday	12 am	Fasting (sleeping)	
	2 am	Fasting (sleeping)	
	4 am	Fasting (sleeping)	
	6 am	Fasting Coffee or tea	
	8 am	Fasting	
	10 am	Fasting	

	12 pm	Lunch: Lasagna (between 12 - 2 pm)	
		Fasting	
	4 pm	Fasting	
	6 pm	Dinner: Cheese and vegetable platter, with sliced turkey or chicken, pickles and olives (between 6 – 8 pm)	
	8 pm	Fasting	
	10 pm	Fasting (sleeping)	
	12 am	Fasting (sleeping)	

Day 5: (12 pm to 8 pm)

Day	Time	Fasting/eating	Exercise
Friday	12 am	Fasting (sleeping)	
	2 am	Fasting (sleeping)	
	4 am	Fasting (sleeping)	
	6 am	Coffee or tea	Jog for 30-60 minutes
	8 am	Fasting	

	Time	Fasting/eating	Exercise
	10 am	Fasting	
	12 pm	Lunch: Boiled eggs with avocado and toast (between 12 - 2 pm)	
	2 pm		
	4 pm		
	6 pm	Dinner (between 6 – 8 pm): Any pasta or Lasagna	
	8 pm	Fasting	Pilates/Yoga class
	10 pm	Fasting (sleeping)	
	12 am	Fasting (sleeping)	

Day 6: (12 pm to 8 pm)

Day	Time	Fasting/eating	Exercise
Saturday	12 am	Fasting (sleeping)	
	2 am	Fasting (sleeping)	
	4 am	Fasting (sleeping)	

	6 am	Fasting Coffee or tea	Jog for 30-60 minutes
	8 am	Fasting	
	10 am	Fasting	
	12 pm	Lunch: Baked salmon with sweet potato (between 12 - 2 pm)	
	2 pm		
	4 pm		Cycling for 1-2 hours
	6 pm	Dinner: Garden salad with stir fried beef or chicken with vegetables (between 6 – 8 pm)	
	8 pm	Fasting	
	10 pm	Fasting (sleeping)	
	12 am	Fasting (sleeping)	

Day 7: (12 pm to 8 pm)

Day	Time	Fasting/eating	Exercise
Sunday	12 am	Fasting (sleeping)	
	2 am	Fasting (sleeping)	
	4 am	Fasting (sleeping)	
	6 am	Coffee or tea	Jog for 30-60 minutes
	8 am	Fasting	
	10 am	Fasting	
	12 pm	Lunch: Baked salmon with arugula and mashed avocado (between 12 - 2 pm)	
	2 pm		
	4 pm		
	6 pm	Dinner: (between 6 – 8 pm) Stir fry chicken or beef with rice and/or salad	
	8 pm	Fasting	Strength training, cardio or yoga class
	10 pm	Fasting (sleeping)	

	12 am	Fasting (sleeping)	

Week 2: 18:6 Fasting

Here, after completing your first week with 16:8 schedule, you'll gradually graduate in week 2 to 18:6. This is an incredibly popular schedule of Intermittent Fasting. It's easy to follow, and even though your fasting hours have increased by 2 hours, you still get enough time to consume two full meals along with a snack in the middle if you like. In the following tables, only breakfast and lunch are presented. You can still have a small snack, like a piece of fruit or green vegetables. You can also consume coffee, tea, water, or bone broth, in your fasting window whenever you see fit.

(Week 2 – Part I)

Day 8: (6 am to 12 pm)

Day	Time	Fasting/eating	Exercise
Monday	12 am	Fasting (sleeping)	
	2 am	Fasting (sleeping)	
	4 am	Fasting (sleeping)	
	6 am	Breakfast: Tea or Coffee, fried eggs, bacon, spinach and toast (between 6 – 8 am)	
	8 am		
	10 am	Early lunch (between 11 am – 12 pm): Platter: olives, cheese, sliced (baked) turkey or chicken, green peppers, cucumbers, etc.	
	12 pm	Fasting	

	2 pm	Fasting	
	4 pm	Fasting	
	6 pm	Fasting	
	8 pm	Fasting	
	10 pm	Fasting (sleeping)	
	12 am	Fasting (sleeping)	

Day 9: (6 am to 12 pm)

Day	Time	Fasting/eating	Exercise
Tuesday	12 am	Fasting (sleeping)	
	2 am	Fasting (sleeping)	
	4 am	Fasting (sleeping)	
	6 am	Breakfast: Coffee or tea, granola cereal with almond, coconut or skim milk (between 6 – 8 am)	Morning run/jog or spin class
	8 am		

	10 am	Early lunch (between 11 am - 12 pm): Shrimp pasta with cream sauce	
	12 pm	Fasting	
	2 pm	Fasting	
	4 pm	Fasting	
	6 pm	Fasting	Weight training/lifting
	8 pm	Fasting	
	10 pm	Fasting (sleeping)	
	12 am	Fasting (sleeping)	

Day 10: (6 am to 12 pm)

Day	Time	Fasting/eating	Exercise
Wednesday	12 am	Fasting (sleeping)	
	2 am	Fasting (sleeping)	

	4 am	Fasting (sleeping)	
	6 am	Breakfast: (between 6 - 8 am): Coffee or tea, avocado, dried basil leaves and tomatoes on toast	Morning run/jog or spin class
	8 am		
	10 am	Early lunch: Eggplant parmesan with pasta (between 11 am - 12 pm)	
	12 pm	Fasting	
	2 pm	Fasting	
	4 pm	Fasting	
	6 pm	Fasting	Weight training/lifting
	8 pm	Fasting	
	10 pm	Fasting (sleeping)	
	12 am	Fasting (sleeping)	

Week 2: Part II

In the second part of week 2, you will follow 18:6 fasting from morning to lunch. Here, your eating window will start from 12 pm and last till 6 pm. The same way as you did previously, you can accommodate lunch and dinner anywhere within your 6 hour eating window, whatever you like. You can have a mid-afternoon snack anywhere between your meals, or you can also choose to pass on that altogether. And because the time for a conventional breakfast falls under your fasting window, you might have tea or coffee or bone broth if you like. Some individuals find it more convenient to pass on breakfast altogether and just enjoy lunch and dinner within their 6 hours of eating window.

Day 11: (12 pm to 6 pm)

Day	Time	Fasting/eating	Exercise
Thursday	12 am	Fasting (sleeping)	
	2 am	Fasting (sleeping)	
	4 am	Fasting (sleeping)	
	6 am	Fasting Coffee or tea	
	8 am	Fasting	
	10 am	Fasting	
	12 pm	Lunch: Fried eggs, bacon, spinach and toast (between 12 – 2 pm)	
	2 pm	Fasting	

	4 pm	Fasting	
	6 pm	Dinner: Platter: olives, cheese, sliced (baked) turkey or chicken, green peppers, cucumbers, etc. (between 4 - 6 pm)	
	8 pm	Fasting	
	10 pm	Fasting (sleeping)	
	12 am	Fasting (sleeping)	

Day 12: (12 pm to 6 pm)

Day	Time	Fasting/eating	Exercise
Friday	12 am	Fasting (sleeping)	
	2 am	Fasting (sleeping)	
	4 am	Fasting (sleeping)	
	6 am	Coffee or tea	Morning run/jog or spin class
	8 am	Fasting	
	10 am	Fasting	

	12 pm	Breakfast: (between 6 – 8 pm) Coffee or tea, granola cereal with almond, coconut or skim milk	
	2 pm		
	4 pm		
	6 pm	Early lunch (between 4 - 6 pm): Shrimp pasta with cream sauce	
	8 pm	Fasting	Weight training/lifting
	10 pm	Fasting (sleeping)	
	12 am	Fasting (sleeping)	

Day 13: (12 pm to 6 pm)

Day	Time	Fasting/eating	Exercise
Saturday	12 am	Fasting (sleeping)	
	2 am	Fasting (sleeping)	
	4 am	Fasting (sleeping)	

	6 am	Coffee or tea	Morning run/jog or spin class
	8 am	Fasting	
	10 am	Fasting	
	12 pm	Lunch: Tea or Coffee, avocado, dried basil leaves and tomatoes on toast (between 12 – 2 pm)	
	2 pm		
	4 pm		
	6 pm	Dinner: (between 6 - 8 pm): Eggplant parmesan with pasta	
	8 pm	Fasting	Weight training/lifting
	10 pm	Fasting (sleeping)	
	12 am	Fasting (sleeping)	

Day 14: (12 pm to 6 pm)

Day	Time	Fasting/eating	Exercise
Sunday	12 am	Fasting (sleeping)	
	2 am	Fasting (sleeping)	
	4 am	Fasting (sleeping)	
	6 am	Fasting	Morning run/jog or spin class
	8 am	Coffee or tea	
	10 am	Fasting	
	12 pm	Lunch: Greek salad with chicken (between 12 - 2 pm)	
	2 pm		
	4 pm		
	6 pm	Dinner: Sushi and miso soup or bone broth (between 4 and 6 pm)	
	8 pm	Fasting	Weight training/lifting
	10 pm	Fasting (sleeping)	

| | 12 am | Fasting (sleeping) | |
| | | | |

Week 3: 18:6 Fasting

The third week will be a continuation of the same eating and fasting windows as week 2. The only difference will be the hours. 18:6 fasting plan will focus on the dinner meal. The eating window begins at 2 pm and until 8 pm. This will work best if you work late or love to have their lunch a bit

later. You can add a quick snack if need be, or shift dinner a bit earlier to have a later snack by 8 pm. You can have bone broth any time in the morning afternoon. If you prefer, you can have bone broth twice while fasting.

Day 15: (2 pm to 8 pm)

Day	Time	Fasting/eating	Exercise
Monday	12 am	Fasting (sleeping)	
	2 am	Fasting (sleeping)	
	4 am	Fasting (sleeping)	
	6 am	Fasting Coffee or tea	
	8 am	Fasting	
	10 am	Fasting Bone broth (optional)	
	12 pm	Fasting	

	2 pm	Lunch: (between 2 – 4 pm) Fried eggs, bacon, spinach and toast	
	4 pm	Fasting	
	6 pm		
	8 pm	Dinner: Platter: olives, cheese, sliced (baked) turkey or chicken, green peppers, cucumbers, etc. (between 6 - 8 pm)	
	10 pm	Fasting (sleeping)	
	12 am	Fasting (sleeping)	

Day 16: (2 pm to 8 pm)

Day	Time	Fasting/eating	Exercise
Tuesday	12 am	Fasting (sleeping)	
	2 am	Fasting (sleeping)	
	4 am	Fasting (sleeping)	
	6 am	Fasting	

	8 am	Coffee or tea	
	10 am	Bone broth	Cycling and/or swimming (60 minutes)
	12 pm	Fasting	
	2 pm	Lunch: Tea or Coffee, crepes or pancakes with fresh fruit and whipped cream (between 2 – 4 pm)	
	4 pm		
	6 pm		
	8 pm	Dinner: Roast beef with sweet potatoes and Brussel sprouts or asparagus(between 6 and 8 pm)	
	10 pm	Fasting (sleeping)	
	12 am	Fasting (sleeping)	

Day 17: (2 pm to 8 pm)

Day	Time	Fasting/eating	Exercise
Wednesday	12 am	Fasting (sleeping)	
	2 am	Fasting (sleeping)	

	4 am	Fasting (sleeping)	
	6 am	Coffee or tea	Morning run/jog or spin class
	8 am	Fasting	
	10 am	Fasting	
	12 pm	Bone broth (optional)	
	2 pm	Mid-day snack/light lunch: Coffee or tea, granola cereal with almond, coconut or skim milk (between 2 -4 pm)	
	4 pm		
	6 pm		Weight training/lifting
	8 pm	Dinner (between 6 and 8 pm): Shrimp pasta with cream sauce	
	10 pm	Fasting (sleeping)	
	12 am	Fasting (sleeping)	

Day 18: (2 pm to 8 pm)

Day	Time	Fasting/eating	Exercise
Thursday	12 am	Fasting (sleeping)	
	2 am	Fasting (sleeping)	
	4 am	Fasting (sleeping)	
	6 am	Coffee or tea	Morning run/jog or spin class
	8 am	Fasting	
	10 am	Fasting	
	12 pm	Bone broth (optional)	
	2 pm	Mid-day snack/light lunch: Boiled eggs with bone broth (between 2 - 4 pm)	
	4 pm		
	6 pm		Any type of cardio
	8 pm	Dinner: Chicken and/or tofu stir fry with vegetables (between 6 - 8 pm)	
	10 pm	Fasting (sleeping)	

| | 12 am | Fasting (sleeping) | |

Day 19: (2 pm to 8 pm)

Day	Time	Fasting/eating	Exercise
Friday	12 am	Fasting (sleeping)	
	2 am	Fasting (sleeping)	
	4 am	Fasting (sleeping)	
	6 am	Fasting (Coffee or tea)	Running/jogging or any type of cardio
	8 am	Fasting	
	10 am	Fasting	
	12 pm	Bone broth (if you want)	
	2 pm	Mid-day snack/light lunch: Coffee or tea, avocado, dried basil leaves and tomatoes on toast (between 2 - 4 pm)	
	4 pm		

	6 pm		Strength training
	8 pm	Dinner: Roast beef with rice noodles and broccoli (between 6 - 8 pm)	
	10 pm	Fasting (sleeping)	
	12 am	Fasting (sleeping)	

Day 20: (2 pm to 8 pm)

Day	Time	Fasting/eating	Exercise
Saturday	12 am	Fasting (sleeping)	
	2 am	Fasting (sleeping)	
	4 am	Fasting (sleeping)	
	6 am	Fasting (Coffee or tea)	Running/jogging or any type of cardio
	8 am	Fasting	
	10 am	Fasting	
	12 pm	Fasting Bone broth (if you like)	

	2 pm	Light lunch: Coffee or tea, Greek yoghurt with berries and granola or chia seeds (between 2 – 4 pm)	
	4 pm		
	6 pm		Any type of cardio
	8 pm	Dinner: Curried chicken and rice or salad(between 6 – 8 pm)	
	10 pm	Fasting (sleeping)	
	12 am	Fasting (sleeping)	

Day 21: (2 pm to 8 pm)

Day	Time	Fasting/eating	Exercise
Sunday	12 am	Fasting (sleeping)	
	2 am	Fasting (sleeping)	
	4 am	Fasting (sleeping)	
	6 am	Fasting	Running/jogging or any type of cardio
	8 am	Fasting (Coffee or tea)	

	10 am	Fasting	
	12 pm	Fasting Bone broth (if you like)	
	2 pm	Light lunch: Grilled cheese with salad (between 12 - 4 pm)	
	4 pm		
	6 pm		Strength training
	8 pm	Dinner: Sushi and miso soup or bone broth (between 6pm - 8pm)	
	10 pm	Fasting (sleeping)	
	12 am	Fasting (sleeping)	

Week 4: 20:4 Fasting

Congratulations on reaching your 4th week. By now, your body has adapted to this eating pattern, and you will be moving to an even bigger fasting window. In your final week, you will transition to 20:4 fasting schedule. It will give you a lot more time to enter autophagy. You also have more flexibility in choosing which 4 hours will consist of your eating window. Usually, 20:4 is comparatively the smallest window after the OMAD (one-meal-a-day) schedule. It will definitely help you to adapt to an even stricter routine like eat stop eat method. This 20:4 routine doesn't allow for two big meals, so only one meal and a quick snack are presented below. Drink a ton of water and bone broth during your fasting window.

Day 22: (6 am to 10 am)

Day	Time	Fasting/eating	Exercise
Monday	12 am	Fasting (sleeping)	
	2 am	Fasting (sleeping)	
	4 am	Fasting (sleeping)	
	6 am	Breakfast: Potato pancakes with sausage or bacon, eggs, Coffee or tea	
	8 am		
	10 am	Mid-morning snack: Banana and berries smoothie	
	12 pm	Fasting	
	2 pm	Fasting	
	4 pm	Fasting	
	6 pm	Fasting	
	8 pm	Fasting	
	10 pm	Fasting (sleeping)	

	12 am	Fasting (sleeping)	

Day 23: (6 am to 10 am)

Day	Time	Fasting/eating	Exercise
Tuesday	12 am	Fasting (sleeping)	
	2 am	Fasting (sleeping)	
	4 am	Fasting (sleeping)	
	6 am	Breakfast: Tea or Coffee, crepes with fresh fruit and whipped cream	Yoga
	8 am		
	10 am	Mid-morning snack: Avocado smoothie	
	12 pm	Fasting	
	2 pm	Fasting	Cycling or swimming
	4 pm	Fasting	

	6 pm	Fasting	
	8 pm	Fasting	
	10 pm	Fasting (sleeping)	
	12 am	Fasting (sleeping)	

Day 24: (6 am to 10 am)

Day	Time	Fasting/eating	Exercise
Wednesday	12 am	Fasting (sleeping)	
	2 am	Fasting (sleeping)	
	4 am	Fasting (sleeping)	
	6 am	Breakfast: Tea or Coffee, scrambled eggs with ham and green peppers	Running/jogging or any type of cardio
	8 am		
	10 am	Mid-morning snack: Avocado smoothie	
	12 pm	Fasting	

	2 pm	Fasting	
	4 pm	Fasting	
	6 pm	Fasting	Pilates/ Yoga session
	8 pm	Fasting	
	10 pm	Fasting (sleeping)	
	12 am	Fasting (sleeping)	

Day 25: (6 am to 10 am)

Day	Time	Fasting/eating	Exercise
Thursday	12 am	Fasting (sleeping)	
	2 am	Fasting (sleeping)	
	4 am	Fasting (sleeping)	
	6 am	Breakfast: Bone broth, tea or Coffee, boiled eggs and	Running/jogging or any type of cardio
	8 am		

	10 am	Mid-morning snack: Smoked tofu with salad	
	12 pm	Fasting	
	2 pm	Fasting	
	4 pm	Fasting	
	6 pm	Fasting	Strength training, cardio and yoga class (60 minutes)
	8 pm	Fasting	
	10 pm	Fasting (sleeping)	
	12 am	Fasting (sleeping)	

Day 26: (6 am to 10 am)

Day	Time	Fasting/eating	Exercise
Friday	12 am	Fasting (sleeping)	
	2 am	Fasting (sleeping)	

	4 am	Fasting (sleeping)	
	6 am	Breakfast: Coffee or tea, Greek yoghurt with berries and granola or chia seeds	Running/jogging or any type of cardio
	8 am		
	10 am	Mid-morning snack: Hummus wrap with vegetables	
	12 pm	Fasting	
	2 pm	Fasting	
	4 pm	Fasting	
	6 pm	Fasting	Strength training, cardio and Pilates class (60 minutes)
	8 pm	Fasting	
	10 pm	Fasting (sleeping)	
	12 am	Fasting (sleeping)	

Day 27: (6 am to 10 am)

Day	Time	Fasting/eating	Exercise
Saturday	12 am	Fasting (sleeping)	
	2 am	Fasting (sleeping)	
	4 am	Fasting (sleeping)	
	6 am	Breakfast: Coffee or tea, poached eggs with bacon and toast	Running/jogging or any type of cardio
	8 am		
	10 am	Mid-morning snack: Avocado and/or cheese	
	12 pm	Fasting	
	2 pm	Fasting	
	4 pm	Fasting	
	6 pm	Fasting	Yoga class
	8 pm	Fasting	

| | 10 pm | Fasting (sleeping) | |
| | 12 am | Fasting (sleeping) | |

Day 28: (6 am to 10 am)

Day	Time	Fasting/eating	Exercise
Sunday	12 am	Fasting (sleeping)	
	2 am	Fasting (sleeping)	
	4 am	Fasting (sleeping)	
	6 am	Breakfast: Coffee or tea, cheese and spinach omelet	Running/jogging or any type of cardio
	8 am		
	10 am	Mid-morning snack: Tuna salad	
	12 pm	Fasting	
	2 pm	Fasting	
	4 pm	Fasting	

	6 pm	Fasting	Strength training, cardio and Pilates class (60 minutes)
	8 pm	Fasting	
	10 pm	Fasting (sleeping)	
	12 am	Fasting (sleeping)	

4.2 Tasty and Healthy Breakfast Recipes

1. Blueberry Pancakes

Preparation Time: 10 minutes

Cooking Time: 10 minutes

Servings: 2

Ingredients:

- 1 cup water
- 1/2 cup icing sugar
- 1 lemon, zest and juice
- 20g butter
- 3 eggs, beaten
- 2 cups frozen blueberries
- 375g pancake mix

Instructions:

- Mix together the eggs and incorporate the sugar.
- Mix in the water and pancake mix well.

- Now incorporate the lemon juice, lemon zest and combine it well.

- Throw in the blueberries and fold the mixture slowly.

- Cook the pancakes with butter until they're golden brown on both sides.

2. Low-Carb Pancake Crepes

Preparation Time: 10 minutes

Cooking Time: 10 minutes

Servings: 2

Ingredients:

- 1 tsp. of cinnamon

- 1 tbsp of sugar-free syrup

- 1 tsp. of almond butter

- 3 oz cream cheese, softened

- 2 eggs, beaten

Instructions:

- Whisk the eggs in a bowl.

- Add the cream cheese, cinnamon, syrup and mix well.

- In a pan melt the butter and fry the pancakes golden brown.

3. Chia Seed Banana Blueberry Delight

Preparation Time: 30 minutes

Cooking time: N/A

Servings: 2

Ingredients

- 1 banana

- 1/4 cup Chia Seeds

- 1 tsp. Vanilla Extract

- 1/2 tsp. Cinnamon

- 1/2 tsp. Salt

- ½ cup blueberries

- 1 cup yogurt

Instructions:

- Remove banana's skin.

- Cut it into medium-thickness circles.

- Then, either mash them up or keep the chunks as they are in case you enjoy it like that.

- Wash the blueberries with water sufficiently.

- Now for 30 minutes or more, soak the chia seeds in water.

- Drain the chia seeds and transfer into a bowl.

- Incorporate the yogurt and combine it all.

- Add the salt, cinnamon and vanilla and mix again.

- Now gently add in blueberries and bananas.

- You can also add some nuts or dried fruit on top right before serving.

- Chill it and enjoy.

4. Egg Omelet

Preparation Time: 10 minutes

Cooking Time: 10 minutes

Serves: 2

Ingredients:

- 2 tbsp butter

- Salt to taste

- 2 tbsp heavy cream

- 1 cup spinach

- ½ tsp. oregano

- 2 sausage, cooked

- Pepper to taste

- 2 eggs

- 1 cup cherry tomatoes

Instructions:

- Chop the cherry tomatoes well.

- Cut the spinach stems. Then cut them into small portions.

- Cut the sausage into thin slices.

- In a skillet, heat up the butter over medium heat.

- With heavy cream in a bowl, beat the eggs and throw the mixture into the skillet.

- Place the egg with oregano, spinach sausage and cherry tomatoes.

- Use some salt and pepper to season.

- Gently fold the omelet.

- Place more oregano on top and serve.

5. Breakfast Muffins

Preparation Time: 10 minutes

Cooking Time: 35 minutes

Serves: 6

Ingredients:

- ½ cup cooked chicken, diced finely

- 2/3 cup coconut flour

- 1 tbsp basil, chopped

- ¼ cup full fat coconut milk

- 1 ½ cup spinach

- ¼ cup diced onion

- ½ tsp. baking powder

- 1 cup shredded cheese

- Salt and pepper to taste

- 8 eggs

Instructions:

- Preheat the oven to 375 degree Fahrenheit.

- Use paper liners or use oil in your muffin tray.

- Beat the eggs in a large mixing bowl.

- Throw in the coconut milk and incorporate well.

- Add in the coconut flour, salt and baking powder.

- Put in the onion, basil, cooked chicken, spinach and mix well.

- Put in the cheese and mix again.

- Transfer this mixture into the muffin tray.

- Bake the muffins in the oven for around 25 minutes.

- Cool it down and serve.

4.3 Tasty and Healthy Lunch Recipes

1. Fish Carrot Potato Salad

Preparation Time: 10 minutes

Cooking Time: 20 minutes

Serves: 2

Ingredients:

- Pepper to taste

- 1 tbsp olive oil

- Salt to taste

- 1 tbsp honey

- 2 small potatoes

- 2-4 radishes

- 1 lemon

- 2 tbsp butter

- Fresh herbs of your choice

- 6-10 green beans

- 2 carrots

- 1 fish fillet of your choice

Instructions:

- Keep the skin and remove the fish bones to give flavor to your salad.

- Heat the oil in a pan over medium high heat.

- Throw in the fish then fry it until it's crispy.

- Move it to the plate.

- Remove the skins from potatoes, radish, and carrots and slice them into long thin sticks.

- Slice the potato and lemon into wedges. Squeeze out 1 tsp. of lemon juice. Use the remaining lemon to garnish.

- Over medium heat, melt the butter in a skillet.

- Gently fry the radish, carrots, sliced potatoes and green beans.

- Transfer all the veggies and fish on a serving plate.

- Garnish with fresh herbs and lemon wedges on top.

- Drizzle some honey and season with salt and pepper. Enjoy!

2. Yellow Squash Soup

Preparation Time: 10 minutes

Cooking Time: 45 minutes

Serves: 6

Ingredients:

- 2 eggs

- 1/3 cup roasted chopped almonds

- 2 garlic cloves, mince

- 1 cup shredded cheese, divided

- ½ cup heavy whipping cream

- 1 onion, chopped

- Salt and pepper to taste

- 1 tsp. butter

- 1 tbsp olive oil

- 4 cups chopped yellow squash

Instructions:

- Preheat the oven to 400 degrees Fahrenheit.

- Use parchment paper to line the baking sheet.

- Place the squash cubes on the baking sheet.

- Grease with oil and season with salt.

- Bake in the oven for no more than 30 minutes.

- Cool it down fully and throw it in the blender. Blend it until a smooth paste emerges.

- Beat the eggs in a pot well.

- Thrown in the squash, butter, garlic, onion and pepper salt.

- Cook for 5 minutes and mix in the cheese and whipping cream.

- Cook again for just 3 minutes.

- Garnish with roasted almonds on top and serve.

3. Spring onion and Sesame Seeds Salmon

Preparation Time: 10 minutes

Cooking Time: 20 minutes

Serves: 4

Ingredients:

- 2 tbsp butter

- 1 tsp. sesame oil

- 1 tsp. onion powder

- 1 tsp. sesame seeds

- 2 tsp. chopped spring onion

- 1 tsp. dried dill weed

- Salt and pepper to taste

- 1 tbsp soy sauce

- 4 salmon fillets

Instructions:

- Pepper, salt, dill and onion powder to season the fish fillets using.

- Marinate it for about half an hour.

- Heat the sesame oil in a pan over medium heat.

- Fry the fish fillets until they become golden in color.

- Move to a plate.

- Melt the butter in the same pan.

- Mix in spring onion and sesame seeds.

- Mix in some soy sauce and cook a minute.

- Pour the sauce on top of the fish. Serve hot.

4. Meatball Soup

Preparation Time: 1 hour

Cooking Time: 25 minutes

Serves: 6

Ingredients:

- 1 tsp. chopped spring onions

- ½ cup sliced onion

- 2 garlic cloves, mince

- Pepper to taste

- 1 tbsp butter

- Fresh herbs of your choice

- 4 cups chicken stock

- 1 tsp. ground ginger

- 1.2 cup soy sauce

- Salt to taste

- 2 pounds ground chicken or turkey

- 2 eggs

Instructions:

- Beat the eggs in a large bowl well.

- Throw in the ground turkey or chicken and incorporate well.

- Mix in some minced garlic, ground ginger, soy sauce and sliced onion.

- Combine everything well and create meatballs with your hands.

- Use plastic wrap to cover the top of the bowl and place it in the fridge.

- Let it sit there for 30 minutes or more.

- Add the chicken stock in a pot.

- Add spring onions, butter and season it with salt and pepper.

- As the stock reach the boiling point, place meatballs gently into the pot.

- Cover it and cook for 10 minutes on medium heat.

- Garnish with herbs and serve hot.

5. Bacon, Lettuce and Tomato Salad

Preparation Time: 5 minutes

Cooking Time: N/A

Serves: 8

Ingredients:

- 2 cups Romaine Lettuce

- 2 cups Iceberg Lettuce

- 2 Chopped scallions

- 2 Diced tomatoes

- 4 Bacon slices

Instructions:

- Mix all of the above-mentioned ingredients.

- Gently put it into a jar.

- Arrange the croutons, veggies and garnish with bacon.

4.4 Tasty and Healthy Dinner Recipes

1. Creamy Chicken Soup

Preparation Time: 15 minutes

Cooking Time: 30 minutes

Serves: 4

Ingredients:

- 1 tsp. lemon juice

- 1 sprig of lemongrass

- Fresh coriander

- 1 green chili

- Salt to taste

- 1 cup milk

- 1 tsp. white pepper

- 1 cube of chicken stock

- 1 tsp. butter

- 1 cup chicken breast, diced

- 1 egg, beaten

Instructions:

- Incorporate everything well in a pressure cooker.

- Close the lid and let it all cook for 10 minutes on low heat.

- Move it all one time and cook again heat for 10 minutes on medium high.

- Serve hot.

2. Vegan Chickpea Burger

Preparation Time: 15 minutes

Cooking Time: 10 minutes

Serves: 2

Ingredients:

- 2 Burger buns
- Salt to taste
- 1 avocado, sliced
- 1 tsp. olive oil
- ½ cup bell pepper, sliced
- 2 lettuce leaves
- 1 onion, diced
- A pinch of white pepper
- A pinch of paprika
- 1 tsp. soy sauce
- 1 tbsp tomato puree
- 1 cup chickpeas, boiled

Instructions:

- Squish the chickpeas and add salt, pepper bell, tomato puree, paprika, pepper and soy sauce.
- Make the mixture into burger patties.
- Fry the patties until they're golden brown on both sides.
- Create a burger by adding onion, lettuce and avocado to the patty and enjoy.

3. Quick Chili

Preparation Time: 10 minutes

Cooking Time: 1 hour

Serves: 4

Ingredients:

- 6 ounce tomato paste
- ½ teaspoon chili powder
- 14 ounce tomato sauce
- 2 cup water or stock
- 3 celery stalks, chopped
- 2 tablespoon oil
- 1 cup diced tomatoes
- 2 tablespoon hot pepper sauce
- 1 cup kidney beans
- 1 cup pumpkin, diced
- ½ cup onion, chopped
- ½ pound lean ground beef

Instructions:

- Put some oil to a pressure cooker and heat it over medium heat.
- Throw in the beef and fry until it's golden brown.
- Move the beef to a plate and add some onion.
- Fry onions until they're golden brown. Then add tomatoes, celery stalk and pumpkin.
- Add the hot pepper sauce and tomato paste and cook for 5 minutes.
- Mix in the beans and stir for about 1 minute.
- Add the fried beef and pour in water or stock.

- Close the lid and cook for 20 minutes on medium heat

- Serve alongside bread or rice or as it is.

4. Cabbage, Egg and Croutons Salad

Preparation Time: 15 minutes

Serves: 2

Ingredients:

- ½ cup torn lettuce

- White pepper to taste

- Salt to taste

- ½ cup Greek Yogurt

- 2 tbsp cheddar cheese

- Any chopped nuts of your choice

- 1 cup cubed cabbage

- 6-8 croutons

- 2 boiled eggs

Instructions:

- Chop each egg into four parts.

- In a large salad bowl, mix in cheddar cheese, pepper and yogurt.

- Add croutons lettuce, eggs, nuts and cabbage and serve.

5. Garlic Chicken Livers

Preparation Time: 10 minutes

Cooking Time: 30 minutes

Serves: 2

Ingredients:

- 4 tablespoon olive oil
- 1 bay leaf
- 1 cup diced onion
- 2 teaspoon lime juice
- 1 cardamom
- Black pepper to taste
- 1 tsp. coriander powder
- 1 tbsp red chili powder
- 1 tbsp ginger garlic paste
- ½ teaspoon salt
- 6 garlic cloves, mince
- 2 tomatoes
- 1 tsp. cumin
- 1 cinnamon stick
- ½ pound chicken liver

Instructions:

- Heat u oil in a large pan over high heat.
- Throw in the garlic and fry until it's golden brown.
- Mix in onion and fry until it's caramelized.
- Put the stove on medium; add cinnamon stick, cardamom and bay leaf. Then mix well for half a minute.

- Add ginger-garlic paste and only 1 tbsp of water to keep it from burning.

- Mix in cumin, salt, black pepper, red chili powder and coriander powder.

- Close the lid and cook for 3 minutes on low heat.

- Mix in chick livers and cook for 15 minutes on medium heat.

- Incorporate tomatoes and cook for another 5 minutes.

- Season it with more salt if necessary.

- Serve hot alongside bread or tortilla.

4.5 Tasty and Healthy Dessert Recipes

1. Frozen Fat Bomb

Preparation Time: 5 minutes

Cooking Time: 2 hours

Serves: 1

Ingredients:

- 1 tsp. Cinnamon

- 1 cup Coconut milk

- 1 tsp. Vanilla extract

- 2 tbsp. Cocoa powder

- 1/4 tsp. Cayenne pepper

- 2 tbsp. Swerve

- 15 drops Stevia

Instructions:

- Begin by checking that the oven is heated up to 400° Fahrenheit.

- In a microwave-safe container, heat up the coconut milk for 20 seconds.

- Mix in the remaining ingredients and incorporate everything well.

- Pour the mixture into an ice cube tray and freeze it for at least 2 hours.

- You can keep the ready cubes in the freezer and consume whenever you like.

2. Crunchy Berry Mousse

Preparation Time: 5 minutes

Cooking Time: 4 hours

Serves: 8

Ingredients:

- Fresh strawberries or blueberries or raspberries (3 oz.)
- 1/4th tsp. vanilla extract
- ½ zested lemon
- 2 oz. chopped pecans
- 2 cups heavy whipping cream

Instructions:

- Whip the cream with a hand mixer until soft peaks appear
- Add the lemon zest and vanilla extract into the whipped cream.
- Gently add in the berries and nuts and mix well.
- Close the bowl's top tightly with some plastic wrap.
- For a sturdier consistency, keep it in the fridge for about four hours.
- You can store it for 3 to 5 days in the fridge. It tastes best on the next day from preparation.

3. Cinnamon Vanilla Bites

Preparation Time: 10 minutes

Cooking Time: 20 - 30 minutes

Serves: 18-20 bites

Ingredients:

- 1/3 cup Quick oats

- ¼ cup Nut butter of choice

- 1 tbsp. Cinnamon

- ¼ cup Pure maple syrup

- ¼ cup Vanilla protein powder

- ½ Almond meal

- 1 tsp. Vanilla extract

Instructions:

- With a layer of parchment paper, cover a cookie tin.

- Process the oats in the food processor and transfer to a mixing bowl. Mix almond meal, cinnamon, nut butter and protein powder.

- Add the vanilla extract and syrup. Now make this dough into small balls.

- Freeze them for 20 to 30 minutes.

- Keep them in a Ziploc container alongside cinnamon and vanilla protein.

- You can keep them in the fridge for as long as 3 weeks and in the freezer for up to six months.

4. Sour Cream Vanilla Cupcake

Preparation Time: 10 minutes

Cooking Time: 20-30 minutes

Serves: 12

Ingredients:

- 4 tbsp. Butter

- 1.5 cups Swerve or any natural sweetener

- 4 Eggs

- 1 tsp. Vanilla

- ¼ cup Sour cream

- 1 cup Almond flour

- ¼ cup Coconut flour

- 1 tsp. Baking powder

- ¼ tsp. Salt

Instructions:

- Preheat your oven to 350° Fahrenheit.

- Mix the butter and sweetener with the electric mixer until they're fluffy and light.

- Mix in the vanilla extract and sour cream. Mix until it's well combined.

- Throw in the eggs one at a time and incorporate well.

- Mix in the flours, salt and baking powder until well combined.

- Pour the batter into 12 muffin cups lined with paper liners.

- Bake for 20-30 minutes or until the cupcakes are firm to the touch and golden brown.

- Cool to room temperature and enjoy.

5. Chocolate Chip Cookie Dough Bites

Preparation Time: 10 minutes

Cooking Time: N/A

Serves: 6

Ingredients:

- 2 tbsp. Butter

- 1 cup Swerve

- 1 tsp. Vanilla extract

- 1.5 oz. Cream cheese

- 1 pinch Sea salt

- ½ cup Sugar-free chocolate chips

Instructions:

- On the medium-low heat setting, mix the sweetener and butter. Cook until they turn thick and light brown in color.

- Now incorporate the vanilla extract and cream cheese well.

- Line a baking tray with wax paper and transfer the mixture onto it.

- Throw the chocolate chips on top of it.

- Put it the fridge to let it set. It can take a day or two. Once it's set, break it into piece and enjoy.

4.6 Tasty and Healthy Snacks Recipes

1. Quick Kale Chips

Preparation Time: 10 minutes

Cooking Time: 10 minutes

Serves: 2

Ingredients:

- Salt as per your taste

- 2 tbsp olive oil

- 1 bunch of kale

Instructions:

- Take of the stem off the kale and rinse them gently a couple of times till they are thoroughly cleaned and ready to be consumed.

- To season the kale, add some salt.

- Cover the baking sheet with a parchment paper in case you wish to bake it.

- Preheat the oven to 170 degrees F.

- On the baking sheet, carefully place the kale pieces and drizzle some olive oil on top.

- Bake it for around 20 minutes.

- If you choose to fry the kale, only fry for 5 minutes and serve hot.

- But if you're baking it, then let it cool to room temperature for 5 minutes and then enjoy.

2. Cheese Chips

Prep time: 5 minutes

Cook time: 10 minutes

Servings: 4

Ingredients:

- Paprika powder, ½ tsp.

- Edam cheese, or provolone cheese or cheddar cheese (shredded) 8 oz.

Instructions:

- Heat up the oven up to 400 degrees Fahrenheit.

- In small heaps, add shredded cheese on a baking sheet lined with foil or parchment paper. Ensure that there is enough distance between them. They must not touch each other.

- Spray Paprika powder on top and bake for eight to ten minutes (depending on the thickness). Be vigilant, so you don't end up burning the cheese because burnt cheese has a bitter taste.

- After baking, remove and place on a cooling rack. Allow to cool and serve.

3. Stilton Eggs

Prep time: 5 – 7 minutes

Cook time: N/A

Servings: 12 pieces

Ingredients:

- 2 tbsp. mayonnaise

- 2 oz. fine Stilton cheese

- 2 tbsp. plain yogurt

- ¼ tsp. salt

- 3 minced green onions

- 6 hard-boiled eggs

- Instructions:

- Peel the eggs and cut them in half.

- Place the whites on a dish and gently put the yolks into a mixing bowl.

- Make a mush of the yolks using a fork. Mix in the yogurt and mayonnaise. Once the yolks become creamy and smooth, add in the Stilton cheese. Leave a few small lumps and mix in the salt and the green onions.

- Put this mixture back into the eggshells.

4. Chicken Wings

Prep time: 10 minutes

Cook time: 60 minutes

Servings: 50 wings

Ingredients:

- 1/2 cup butter

- 2 tsp. paprika

- 1 tbsp. dried oregano

- 4 pounds chicken wings

- 1 cup grated Parmesan cheese

- 1 tsp. salt

- 2 tbsp. dried parsley

- 1/2 tsp. pepper

Instructions:

- Preheat the oven to 350° Fahrenheit.

- Cut the wings into drumsticks and keep the pointy tips. If you're wondering what to do with wingtips, freeze them for soup; they'll make a good broth.

- In a bowl, mix the parsley, oregano, paprika, parmesan cheese, pepper and salt.

- Cover a shallow baking pan on the inside with foil. Skipping this will leave stubborn marks on your pan.

- Take a shallow bowl or pan and melt the butter.

- Cover all drumsticks in butter, then roll in the seasoning and cheese concoction, and place in the baking pan.

- Bake them for 1 hour and serve hot.

5. Bacon Cheeseburger Bites

Prep time: 5 minutes

Cook time: 60 minutes

Servings: 6

Ingredients:

- Salt

- 12 oz. ground beef

- ½ tsp. garlic powder

- Black pepper

- ½ cup diced yellow onion

- 12 slices raw bacon

Instructions:

- Preheat your oven to 350° Fahrenheit. Cover a baking sheet with foil.

- Mix the ground beef with garlic powder, salt, onion and pepper.

- Make twelve beef balls.

- Wrap each beef ball in a bacon slice and arrange on the baking pan.

- Bake for 60 minutes until the bacon becomes crispy.

Conclusion

Thank you for reading through to the end of *Intermittent Fasting for Women After 50*. By now, you must've found this book to be extremely helpful in providing you with all of the resources you need to accomplish your health and longevity goals, whatever they might look like for you.

Now, the next step in your health journey is to move further and decide on a plan you'll follow that can catapult you to a higher degree of success. If you do need assistance getting underway, you'll probably get great results by first reviewing your daily diet and exercise routine before deciding on a feasible intermittent fasting regimen. Remember, you're not bettering your health for others; you're doing it for yourself future. Intermittent fasting is a fantastic way to schedule meal hours, not just for losing fat but also for leading a healthy, vibrant lifestyle that has many health benefits.

Considering how busy life is for women of any age, intermittent fasting, specifically for older women, is unlike all the other weight-loss plans, which are either very hard to follow every day consistently, are costly, and produce just modest results. Intermittent fasting is both free and quick to enforce. Simply alter your dietary habits such that you alternate times of fasting with periods of feasting. This book is a particularly valuable guide for helping you during the adjustment to a new way of life. Know you don't have to alter your diet; alternatively, adopt a different form of eating that suits your lifestyle. In fact, you could still carry on with your exercise program even though you'll have to customize it to the existing scenario in contexts of when you consume food and how intense your gym sessions are.

So, what exactly are you looking for? Start planning for your intermittent fasting journey now to enjoy the rewards. Use the knowledge you've gained from this book as a launching pad to get ready for and change your life.

Of course, a healthy lifestyle has many forms: it doesn't look the same for everyone. Intermittent fasting is just one of the many amazing options people have to better one's health. The most essentials and central tenets of any good lifestyle are still going to be consuming natural, organic food, staying active, and improving your sleep quality. Intermittent fasting can be challenging in the beginning. So if intermittent is not your cup of tea even after trying hard, then you can surely keep looking for the lifestyle that best suits your life and goals and is feasible for you. Because when all is said and done, there is no one-size-fits-all diet or lifestyle when it comes to your longevity and fitness. The best plan is the one that you can sustain for a lifetime. Consistency is everything in life. If you feel at your best during your fasts and find it to be a maintainable way of living, it can be like magic for you to lose weight and improve your health.

If you enjoyed the book, let me know what you thought by leaving me a review on Amazon.

Thanks,

Martha Kirby